For anyone who has ever felt “off” and couldn’t find the words to explain it.

For those navigating bloating, burnout, brain fog, or being dismissed.

This is your validation. This is your roadmap. This is your reset.

—

For my children, and for those I’ve been blessed to love and guide along the way.

The next generation of Forward ThinKers.

May you always trust your body, your heart, and your purpose.

With love and light <3

Foreword

"Jackie Frary offers a truly holistic view of gut health, one that honors our connection to ourselves, to our rhythms, and to others. Her approach is engaging, clear, and hopeful."

— Cindy Geyer, MD, The UltraWellness Center, Berkshires, MA

"I am so thankful to have had Jackie in my life during my gut-healing journey. It can be a lonely process, and Jackie was always supportive, caring, and full of light.

I would often share new information I discovered, and she would meet me with her knowledge, encouragement, and insight. Her passion for living well inspired me and helped me along my own path to healing."

— DF, Merrimack, NH

Acknowledgments

Without the individuals, professionals, and events that influenced my recovery, this book would not have been possible.

To **Dr. Mark Hyman, MD, Dr. Cynthia Geyer, MD, Annette Quatrano,** and the entire team at The UltraWellness Center—thank you for validating my symptoms, listening deeply, and helping me piece together a body I once thought was permanently broken.

To **Yvonne Fulciniti**, who crossed my path at just the right moment and set me on the testing journey that changed everything—thank you for your grounded wisdom and spark of divine timing.

To the countless people I've coached, chatted with, and traded healing stories with—**you helped me make sense of my own experience by reflecting your truth back to me**. Thank you for your vulnerability and trust.

A special thank-you to **Veronica St. Cyr**, whose creative eye and calming presence helped bring my vision to life. From the website to the book cover, your design, dedication, and heart helped shape the soul of this project.

To my incredible family—thank you for your prayers, your patience, your laughter, and your willingness to go "glutton-free" even when it wasn't easy. Your love reminded me what wholeness feels like.

And to the quiet faith that guided me when I had nothing left but trust—thank you, God, for carrying me through.

To my body—thank you for never giving up on me, even when I didn't understand you.

And to every person reading this who feels like they've "tried it all"—**you're not crazy, you're not weak, and you're absolutely not alone.** May this book be your reminder and your roadmap.

Preface

Why Gut Healing Matters

At some point, we stop asking, *"What's wrong with me?"* and start asking, *"What's my body trying to tell me?"*

That question changed my life. It led me through skin rashes, food reactions, endless Google searches, years of trial and error—and, eventually, to a new blueprint for living. One rooted in truth, transformation, and trust in the healing intelligence of the body.

This book was born out of that journey.

I didn't write this because I have a degree behind my name. I wrote it because I lived it. I lived the confusion. I lived the inflammation. I lived the frustration of being told, "Your labs look fine," while my body was screaming otherwise.

Before the Breakthrough

I was exhausted—but wired. Bloated—but underweight. Breaking out in rashes but just being handed tubes and jars of expensive creams. Deep down, I knew something was wrong. And no prescription was addressing the root.

It wasn't until I discovered the **gut-brain connection**—and met functional medicine practitioners who helped me connect the dots—that my healing began.

I wish I'd had this book when I was at my lowest. It's half science, part spirit, and part protocol. It brings together scientific knowledge, spiritual guidance, and practical guidelines, all with heart and given with sincere intent. Traditional medicine and functional medicine both have their place. Lab testing, prescriptions, and emergency care save lives every day. What I learned on my own journey is that true healing happens when you bridge the two, using traditional medicine for diagnosis and choosing holistic tools for rebuilding balance and prevention. My intention is to hand you hope, backed by evidence and results.

This book was written with deep care, but not perfection. If you find a typo or two, consider it part of the proof that real life, like real healing, is never flawless. I wrote this as a guide who has walked through the fire. I know what it's like to feel like you're doing everything right yet still feel wrong inside. To have doctors dismiss your symptoms. To carry invisible discomfort for so long that it starts to feel normal. But this is not normal. And it is not your fault.

The Internal Fungus Among Us is your roadmap back to balance. It's built from research, resilience, and a protocol that works—one I've tested, lived, and refined. In these pages, we'll explore the hidden link between your gut and your mind, how stress and trauma disrupt your biology, and how you can heal with food, breath, movement, and mindset.

If you're tired of quick fixes, done feeling dismissed, and finally ready to feel like yourself again, this book is for you.

Healing is not a straight line. But with the right support, the right questions, and the right plan, healing is possible.

Author's Note

I know what it's like to feel dismissed, bloated, exhausted—like your body is a mystery even the experts can't solve. I've been there: in the fog of fatigue, with supplements on the counter and no real answers in sight.

You don't need more advice. You need a roadmap that honors your intuition. A healing path that includes your mind, your story, and your spirit—not just your symptoms. In these pages, you'll find more than protocols.

You'll find permission: To slow down. To listen inward. To question everything. And to finally trust your gut, in more ways than one. Whether you're just starting or already halfway there, I want this book to feel like a hand on your back and a voice that reassures you: "You're not broken. You're becoming. Let's walk this together."

There is a divine strength in surrender—not giving up but giving it over.

— Jackie Frary

Introduction

I always thought that when I finally wrote a book, I'd start from the end. Maybe I'm just impatient, or maybe I'm a no-nonsense kind of woman who likes to get straight to the point. So here it is: I am now a healthy woman in my early fifties. Vibrant. Clear headed. Grounded. But it wasn't always this way.

A Girl from "The County"

I grew up on a farm in the deep, northern woods of Maine—"The County," as we call it. My childhood was filled with fresh air, frozen winters, endless summers, and lots of movement. I climbed ropes to the top of the gymnasium like it was nothing. Ran track like the wind. I was strong and capable and didn't know how not to be.

We ate meat, potatoes, and rarely anything processed. I knew even then that cereal and milk didn't sit well with me. Every morning before school, that combo left me nauseated and cramping. By the time I got on the school bus, my stomach felt like it was doing backflips. Going to the bathroom became a guessing game. And that's where my gut journey began—quiet, invisible, and totally misunderstood.

As the youngest of five kids, I was always out to prove myself. I grew up fast. "Adulting" started early for me. I worked three jobs and still made time for fun. I stayed up late, fueled by what today's generation calls FOMO—"fear of missing out." I didn't know the term back then, but trust me, I had it down to an art form. My foot was always on the gas.

As a result, most of my adult life was spent fighting a battle I didn't even know I was in.

Brain fog. Irritability. Crippling bloating. Cramps that knocked the wind out of me. Joint pain that made me feel twice my age. The list grew over time, and so did my frustration. Doctors offered creams, pills, and the occasional shrug. The root cause? It took me decades to discover I was battling an **internal imbalance**: **candidiasis** (fungal infection from yeast overgrowth), **SIBO** (small intestinal bacteria overgrowth), **IBS** (irritable bowel syndrome), and **chronic constipation**. This was an ecosystem inside me gone *rogue*. A silent, systemic inflammation with deep roots in the gut.

Like so many others, I learned to hide it. I masked the pain with physical activity, warm compresses, and mental toughness. I kept moving. That was my thing—motion over emotion. But when I look back, the signs were there all along.

What You'll Find Inside

This is not just another gut book. It's a roadmap for resetting your body and mind through:

- **Functional nutrition** that works with your symptoms and lifestyle
- **Supplements and detox tools** that support your unique biochemistry
- **Movement and emotional release practices** that heal more than just your digestion
- **Real-life protocols**, grocery guides, and insights from the front lines of recovery

Whether you're dealing with *Candida* overgrowth, SIBO, IBS, anxiety, fatigue, or "mystery symptoms" your doctor can't explain, you are not alone.

How This Book Is Structured

Each chapter builds upon the last to guide you through a full-body healing reset:

1. Understand the **gut-brain connection**.
2. Learn how **stress, trauma, and food** create inflammation.
3. Rebuild your health with **customized protocols**.
4. Anchor your new vitality with **lifestyle tools and mindset shifts**.
5. Take action with your **30-day reset plan** resources.

This book combines expert-backed strategies from leaders like **Dr. Mark Hyman, MD,** and **Cynthia Geyer, MD**, as well as the wisdom of integrative nutrition and my own lived experience of reversing chronic symptoms.

Chapter 1: The Gut-Brain Connection

How Your Gut Talks to Your Brain and Why It Changes Everything

Throughout this book, I'll be talking about "the gut." This is, specifically, the body's entire digestive system—from the "in" all the way to the "out." It includes, among other neighboring parts, the stomach, small and large intestines, intestinal lining, and the many organisms working in those spaces to help you digest food and absorb nutrients.

The gut-brain axis is a superhighway that connects your digestive system and your brain. Recent research on the gut-brain axis shows that everything you eat, every stress you feel, and every emotion you show or hide can affect the complicated interactions in your stomach. And here's where it gets interesting: your gut and brain are always talking to each other, like some old married couple. One barks instructions, and the other responds. One gets mad, and the other feels it right away. The relationship is close and direct, and it affects both physical and mental health.

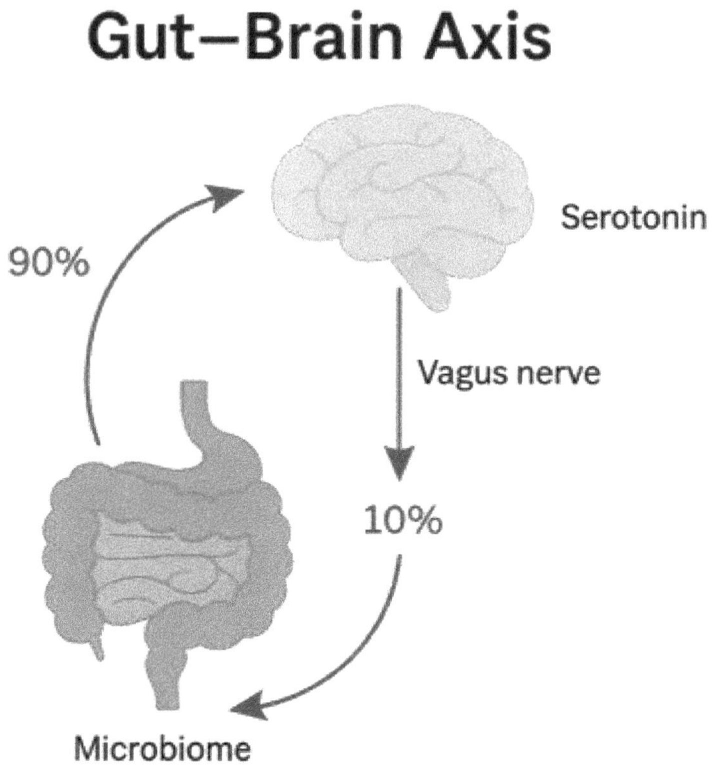

Learning about the gut-brain link helped me figure out what was really wrong with my health, which led to a more complete approach to my health. Functional medicine helped me find the fundamental issues, while traditional medicine gave me the tests, labs, and safety net I needed along the road. I never had to choose a side. Both kinds of medicine had their own knowledge, and the secret was using them together.

It's Not "All in Your Head"—It's Also in Your Gut

Have you ever felt "butterflies" before a big meeting? Lost your appetite when you were sad? Had to run to the bathroom when anxiety hit?

That's not a coincidence. It's what people frequently call the "second brain." It sends signals, reacts to stress, and affects everything from mood to immunity. I learned that your gut makes more than 90% of the body's serotonin, which controls mood, sleep, and emotions.

So your gut isn't just a "plumbing" system; it's a whole command center doing far more than most of us were ever taught.

The Microbiome: Your Internal Ecosystem

Inside your gut lives a bustling city of microbes, bacteria, fungi, and viruses—more than 100 trillion organisms working around the clock. This collection is called your microbiome, and it's as unique to you as your fingerprint.

Most people don't know that *Candida* and other fungi living in your gut aren't "bad." *Candida albicans* is a natural yeast that lives on and in our body. It's supposed to be there. When your gut is healthy, it actually helps protect you from other pathogens. The problem starts when *Candida* grows faster than your body can keep in check. Because yeasts are a type of fungus, an overproduction of *Candida* is problematic.

And that's exactly what happened to me. My gut stopped being a garden and started to look more like an overrun field. Stress, antibiotics, sugar, exhaustion, and pushing through instead of slowing down all merged to create the perfect storm. The good bacteria got smaller, the fungi grew too much, and my whole system felt like it was turning against me.

When the microbiome is thrown off like that, whether it's because of lifestyle, trauma, nutrition, or just years of ignoring the whispers, everything spirals. It's like a garden. Stop tending it, and the weeds move in. And in my situation, those weeds had taken over everything. This kind of disruption can look like this:

- Bloating and cramping
- Brain fog and fatigue
- Skin issues like rashes or acne
- Joint pain and inflammation
- Anxiety and depression
- Sugar cravings that feel impossible to resist

These symptoms aren't simply in your brain; they could mean your body is inflamed. And it wasn't just my body that broke down.

My Breaking Point Wasn't Just Physical

When I first heard the term *gut-brain axis*, I didn't know whether to roll my eyes or cry with relief. Finally, something made sense of why I felt so bad and why nothing conventional seemed to help.

I used to think my symptoms were unrelated: stomach issues on one hand, mood swings and fatigue on the other. I had no idea they were all part of the same web, with the same core problem showing up in different systems.

I was functioning, but I wasn't thriving. That was the moment that changed everything for me. I was tired of patching leaks; I wanted to rebuild the foundation.

The Gut-Brain Axis Is Your Healing Highway

Your gut-brain axis is your internal highway—and whether you're speeding, stalled, or rerouted by inflammation, it can be recalibrated.

Author and podcast host Mel Robbins calls this "The Power of The Pause." That reminder—to slow down, reset, and return to self—became a guiding principle for me. I'm grateful for her work and her influence on my journey.

When Science Meets Experience

Holistic healers have known for a long time that taking care of your gut health is good for your mental health. We're seeing more and more proof of this point. Researchers using the NIH library of medicine and PubMed have found that a greater variety of microbiome and healthier gut-microbe communities are linked to lower rates of anxiety and depression and, possibly, better responses to stress. Some studies on people and animals given probiotics and prebiotics have even shown lower amounts of cortisol (the stress hormone) and signs of better resilience to stress and trauma. Though research is still in its early stages, combining gut-healthy lifestyle choices with common mental-health treatments is a strong way to start healing.

I'm not a scientist (and I don't pretend to be), but I did a lot of study and worked with specialists to learn about the gut-brain link. What you'll read here isn't theory from a lab; it's lived experience supported by the best evidence I could find.

But the truth is that healing is a personal path that is different for everyone based on their own past and situation. Your history, habits, stress level, and the specific microbial fingerprint of your gut all affect how you heal. This book offers a flexible framework, allowing you to adapt its insights to your unique healing journey.

Why This Chapter Matters

Before we talk about protocols and plans, supplements and superfoods, we need to do one very crucial thing:

- Conceptually reconnect your gut and your brain.
- Believe they belong together.

- Understand that healing one heals the other.

Let's bring you back into balance. You are not broken—you're just misaligned. And soon you'll discover how to reset the system from the inside out.

Coming Up Next

In the next chapter, I'll take you deeper into my personal transformation—what it took to go from barely holding it together to living with clarity, calm, and vitality. I'll share what worked, what didn't, and why healing your gut isn't just about food—it's about listening to the messages your body has been trying to send you all along.

Notes

HealthGarden. (n.d.). "Frequently Asked Questions." healthgardenusa.com/pages/faqs. Accessed December 6, 2025.

You Are What You Eat. "Eat for a Happier Mind: How Nutrition Affects Mental Health." mywayofhealth.com/blog/eat-for-a-happier-mind-how-nutrition-affects-mental-health. Published May 20, 2025.

Chapter 2: My Story, Rock Bottom to Rebuild

From Fungus to Freedom

If you're anything like me, you've probably been dismissed, misdiagnosed, and given advice that didn't really help. The advice I got didn't work because I kept going to the same source (the doctor) for the same problems. I needed to look more closely at what was really going on with me. What I'm sharing isn't just a story; it's a guide. What happened to me isn't rare; it's just not talked about very often with this much honesty.

First, let's go back.

From Strong to Stalled

I was always in good shape. I grew up on a farm in northern Maine, where I was a girl who could outrun the boys and climb to the top of the rope in gym class. I was strong, fast, and active. But even though I looked healthy on the outside, something was wrong on the inside.

I was 19 when I noticed the rash. My shoulders, blotchy and red. I thought maybe it was from a tanning bed. The doctor said it was a fungal infection. "Here's a cream—apply it for seven to ten days," he said. That was the first of dozens of prescriptions I'd receive over the next few decades. The rash came back every year like clockwork. And every year, I applied and reapplied, never once realizing this was a symptom, not the cause.

By my thirties, I was married with kids and managing a demanding career in media sales. I met celebrities, attended concerts, and lived a big life with my kids in tow. I made unforgettable memories. But high performance came at a cost. The stress was constant. My sleep was shallow. Still, I kept going.

I had an "I've got this" attitude. But under the surface, my body was waving the white flag, trying to get a message through to me. I lived with:

- Brain fog
- Bloating and cramps
- Rashes that wouldn't go away
- Constipation
- Painful joints
- Irritability and fatigue

Doctors would often say these recurring symptoms were "just stress," but I knew better than that. My body was whispering long before it started to scream.

The Silent Invaders: *Candida*, SIBO, and IBS

At one point, I was told that the rash on my shoulders was just a basic fungal problem. I used creams for years, not knowing they were treating only a small part of a bigger problem: *Candida* overgrowth—the "good guys" gone bad. I was sitting by a campfire one minute, and the next minute the camp was on fire. That might sound a little dramatic, but that's how *Candida* overgrowth felt in my body.

I eventually learned that I also have SIBO, or small intestinal bacterial overgrowth. This means there is too much bacteria in my small intestine. SIBO can make you feel bloated; give you gas, stomach pain, and diarrhea; and make it hard for your body to absorb nutrients. Did you catch that? *Trouble absorbing nutrients*. Thinking about this right now hurts me. My intestines had one job, but they couldn't do it because my body wouldn't let them. Then came SIBO's best friend, irritable bowel syndrome (IBS), which is not surprising, since the two go hand in hand. All of these were signs that something had taken over my gut!

What's wild is this: I was doing everything "right." I ate clean, took supplements, and worked out, but I was still inflamed, bloated, and stuck.

That's when I met Yvonne Fulciniti, CHHC, AADP, a Certified Holistic Health Coach, in a health food store. We talked for over an hour. While I was waiting to see Dr. Mark Hyman at the UltraWellness Center, she recommended I get a food sensitivity test.

At that point, I had already cleared my rash by playing health detective—rotating protocols, trying out herbs and supplements, cutting out certain foods (including some fun foods/beverages), and learning about functional medicine. I studied health and nutrition, as well as Ayurvedic practices. I learned the science. I worked out. I looked on the internet and found Dr. Hyman's 10-day detox. I was making progress. But I needed some order and a baseline. I had already been through so much and needed to keep going. I needed a medical team to help me keep the monster at bay.

The Turning Point: Functional Medicine, Data, and Determination

Everything shifted when I began working with Cynthia Geyer, MD, at the UltraWellness Center.

Her method was thorough, caring, and tailored to each patient. Instead of writing off my symptoms, she looked into them more.

- Ordered GI Effects testing, NutrEval, and genetic testing
- Looked at my calcium metabolism (how calcium is broken down) because I've had kidney stones

- Investigated my hormones, my body's stress response, and the permeability of my gastrointestinal tract
- Identified high yeast markers, low butyrate, and dysbiosis (microbial imbalance)

She confirmed what I had long suspected: my microbiome was out of whack, my nervous system was under stress, and my digestion wasn't just slow; it was out of balance.

My Custom Protocol: A Three-Month Reset Plan

Getting to action items is fun for me, and, frankly, this beast was a second job, so embracing action items brought me peace.

Based on what Dr. Geyer and dietitian Annette Quatrano told us, we came up with a multi-phase healing plan.

- Targeted supplementation
- Finding the root causes through lab tests
- Changes in my lifestyle
- A fresh start for my whole body

Here's a quick look at the process that made everything different:

Mind-Body Connection

- Meditation and breathing exercises (starting with Deepak Chopra's 21-Day Series)
- Cortisol Manager for stress-related insomnia
- Daily walks, weight training, and resistance workouts (eGym)

Core Supplements

- **Biocidin**: Five drops three times a day to get rid of yeast and biofilm in my intestines.

- **Seed probiotics**: Two capsules every day, one in the morning and one at night to help get things rebalanced
- **Motility Activator** (ginger and artichoke blend) to help my bowel movements
- **Turmeric digestive bitters** before meals to help my stomach
- **Evening primrose oil** for my skin, hormones, and omega-6 levels
- **Magnesium citrate**: 400 mg in the morning to help my bowel movements
- **Magnesium glycinate**: 400 mg at night to help me relax
- **K-Force (Vitamin D3 + K2)** for my immune system, hormones, and bones
- **BCAA powder** to help my muscles recover after strength training
- **DHEA** (10 mg) to help with adrenal fatigue and menopausal changes

They were added carefully, monitored closely, and changed when they needed to be. It took a long time, but I wouldn't change it.

The Nutrition Plan: Fighting *Candida*, Reviving Me

Yes, I was doing a lot of good things, but how do you know whether you're doing everything right? For example, I thought eggs were a great source of protein for me, besides being a quick and easy breakfast option. I had no idea eggs were making my body inflamed.

Based on my food sensitivity test and GI results, Annette helped me make a nutrition plan that would heal my gut, put out the fire, and balance my hormones.

- **Gluten free, dairy free, egg free, and low carb**

- **Protein-first:** starting every meal with protein (plant + animal combo)
- **Healthy fats:** ghee, nuts, seeds, avocado, omega-3s
- **Smart carbs:** quinoa, lentils, root veggies, moderate amounts of fruit
- **Fermented and prebiotic foods (as tolerated):** asparagus, onions, chickpeas, green bananas
- **Detox support:** cruciferous veggies, clean water, sweating often
- **Low oxalates:** boiling greens, soaking beans, avoiding excess spinach/chocolate

My meals became medicine—not just restriction.

Symptoms Transformed

Here's what changed after I followed this plan:

- **Bloating**
  Then: Daily
  Now: Occasionally, with known triggers
- **Constipation**
  Then: Lifelong struggle
  Now: Rarely, thanks to probiotics
- ***Candida* rash**
  Then: Recurring
  Now: Gone (occasional known flare-up)
- **Fatigue**
  Then: Persistent
  Now: Stable and strong energy level
- **Mood and Focus**
  Then: Irritable, foggy
  Now: Clear, calm, grounded
- **Sleep**
  Then: Interrupted

Now: Deep, fairly consistent (especially with cortisol manager)

- **Joint Pain**
  Then: Nagging
  Now: Gone

Relapses Happen—But I Have the Tools

My candidiasis got worse after I came into contact with mold in 2023. But this time I was ready and had my tools. Even though I wasn't happy about it, I did the work, did the research, and yes, it was a lot, but I knew what to do:

- **Restore my gut** with digestive bitters, reduced stress, and lower fruit/sugar intake
- **Support my liver** with activated charcoal and reintroducing Berberine, Triphala, and milk thistle
- **Reset my lifestyle** with increased sunlight and movement, probiotics, oregano oil, garlic, pau d'Arco tea

I used the experience as a *reset,* not a setback. Because true healing isn't linear. It's a spiral—every loop brings you closer to yourself.

Why Your Story Starts Here

I'm not looking for sympathy when I tell my story. I want to help someone, or many people, who are going through the fire. I want to give you the tools I gained so you can get a head start on where you are and what you're going through right now. If you've felt dismissed, confused, or stuck in your symptoms—you're not alone. You're not damaged. And you don't need another generic fix.

I hope you can take everything I learned from my process and use it as a guide to look back on when you're spinning. You deserve answers, someone who has been there to help you on your personal journey to find what you need to get to the other side.

Coming Up Next

Now that you've begun to understand how your gut and brain affect each other, I want to tell you how this science worked out for me. There is a story behind every symptom, and mine began long before I knew what *Candida* was.

Notes

The Gut Health Dietician. "What are the Signs of SIBO I Might be Ignoring?" guthealthdietitian.com/blog/SIBO. Accessed December 6, 2025.

Chapter 3: The Modern Gut Crisis

Why We're More Inflamed, Intolerant, and Imbalanced Than Ever

Let's be honest: your gut was never designed to digest stress, ultra-processed food, chronic multitasking, and social media doomscrolling—all before noon. And yet, that's become our modern routine.

We wake up every day to a cup of coffee and rush of cortisol. We scroll past headlines that spike our nervous systems before we've even had water. We rush out the door, grabbing "food" engineered to sit on a shelf longer than it would last in our bodies. Then we wonder why we feel foggy, inflamed, reactive, exhausted, and stuck.

It's not your imagination. You are more than simply "getting older." You're living in what I call "The Modern Gut Crisis."

The Real Epidemic: Disconnection

This crisis isn't just biological—it's cultural. We're living in a state of disconnection:

- From our bodies
- From seasonal rhythms
- From food grown in soil
- From the signals within ourselves

And sadly, more people are disconnected from each other. We were not made to live in silos. Instead, we're plugged into fast food, faster lifestyles, and medical systems that too often address symptoms, not root causes.

This is what we're truly up against:

Overuse of Antibiotics

The Centers for Disease Control and Prevention (CDC) believes that at least one out of every three antibiotic prescriptions in U.S. outpatient settings, such as doctors' offices and emergency rooms, are not needed. [1] These powerful medications can save lives, but they can also wipe out healthy gut flora along with the bad stuff if you don't actually need them. This can cause an imbalance of microbes in the gut and lead to infections, including *Candida* overgrowth.

Ultra-Processed Diets

According to the CDC, ultra-processed foods make up around 55% of the calories eaten by Americans who are 1 year old or older (2021–2023).[1] Even though definitions range, these foods frequently have processed sugars, artificial sweeteners, dyes, highly refined oils, and other industrial ingredients in them. These are completely different from the whole foods that are healthiest for your body and help your gut repair.

Chronic Stress

The stress hormone cortisol slows motility (movement of food and waste through the digestive system), decreases important stomach acid, and makes the immune system in the mucous membranes weaker—a recipe for bloating, constipation, and gut inflammation.

Stress also depletes magnesium and B vitamins, which are both crucial for creating neurotransmitters and mending the digestive system. (I know this lack of "B" firsthand from when my doctor was giving me shots where the sun doesn't shine.)

Many of us aren't "just tired"—we're living in a constant state of fight-or-flight.

Environmental Toxins

We're all exposed to more environmental stuff than our grandparents ever were—pesticides on our food, chemicals in plastics, heavy metals in water, even mold hiding in our homes. It sounds intense, but here's the part I want you to hear: you don't have to panic about any of this. I didn't write this to scare you. I wrote it because understanding what touches your body helps you understand what your body might be trying to tell you.

Some of these exposures may harm the gut lining and microbiome over time, especially if your body is already stressed or overburdened. That was me for a long time, to be honest. I pushed through and ignored the signs, not realizing how much my gut was attempting to keep up with.

What about "leaky gut"? This rising term may sound like a trendy phrase, but it's far more common than people realize. Increased intestinal permeability is a real, medically recognized process that shows up in research around inflammation, allergies, autoimmune issues, and chronic stress. When your gut lining gets irritated or overwhelmed, your whole body can feel it.

Truth is you can't heal from things you don't know. And that's part of the story—yours and mine. But here's where the story changes, there's hope in all of this:

Your gut can heal.

It responds to care, rest, and nourishment in ways that still amaze me. You don't have to fix everything at once or become the cleanest eater on the planet. Little shifts create big changes over time. I'm living proof of that.

I love a happy ending, and there is a way.

Low-Fiber, Low-Color Diets

Fiber is fuel for your good gut bacteria, especially the soluble, plant-based prebiotics that nourish your microbiome. Plates that are mostly beige (think white bread, pasta, minimal veggies) don't give your gut the color, variety, and nourishment it needs to thrive.

Gut Impact, Brain Fallout

Let's get one thing straight: what happens in the gut *does not* stay in the gut.

Your gut is the foundation of your immune system, your mood, your hormones, and your ability to think clearly.

Do any of these symptoms sound familiar?

- Brain fog
- Afternoon crashes
- Bloating after "healthy" meals
- Insomnia or waking at 3 a.m.
- Mood swings or irritability
- Chronic itching or breakouts
- Sugar cravings that feel like sabotage

These aren't random. They're signals. Your gut is trying to tell you something, and the longer you ignore it, the louder the signals get.

A disrupted microbiome affects:

- **Mood and Mental Health:** Ninety percent of serotonin (one of the body's "feel-good" chemicals) is produced in the gut. Imbalanced micbrobes = unstable emotions.

- **Cognition:** When your gut isn't absorbing nutrients well and your neural tissue is inflamed, you can end up with brain fog and memory issues.
- **Hormones:** Your body's ability to break down and remove excess estrogen depends on a healthy gut-liver axis (think PMS, PCOS, and menopause symptoms).
- **Autoimmunity:** Leaky gut contributes to inflammation throughout the body and to immune system misfires.
- **Skin Conditions:** Acne, eczema, and rashes often trace back to an imbalance of microbes in the gut.

This Is Not Your Fault

Here's the truth: you didn't create this mess. It was inherited—from a culture, a food system, and even a medical model that doesn't always ask *why*. I want to make it clear that traditional medicine is very important. It gives life-saving treatments, tests, and important information. Personally, I never had a problem with medicine itself; I had a problem with the time between appointments when my symptoms got worse. Functional medicine helped me fill in the gaps, but it didn't take the place of my doctor.

Functional medicine offers a different lens, one that sees the body not as broken, but as beautifully intelligent and constantly seeking balance.

> "Everything shifted when I began working with Dr. Cynthia Geyer at Dr. Hyman's UltraWellness Center."

That single sentence was the turning point in my own story. From years of experimenting, eliminating, journaling, and managing symptoms on my own, I stepped into partnership with a team who saw my full picture—who treated the terrain, not just the symptoms.

That's when healing deepened, and I could finally exhale.

Notes

[1] Centers for Disease Control and Prevention. "About 30 percent of antibiotics prescribed in the outpatient setting are unnecessary." CDC Newsroom, May 3, 2016.

[2] Centers for Disease Control and Prevention. *What We Eat in America: Consumption of Ultra-Processed Foods Among U.S. Children and Adults, 2021–2023.* NHANES, published 2024.

Coming Up Next

The gut is the gateway. It is the mediator between your inner and outer world—between nourishment and inflammation, depletion and restoration.

In the next chapter, we'll explore the gut-brain connection, the role of stress and trauma in gut dysfunction, and why learning to regulate your nervous system is just as important as your probiotic routine.

The path to healing begins with awareness. And awareness begins right here.

Author's Reflection

While my journey may sound personal, it's also painfully common. We're not just dealing with one broken body—we're living through a broken system. Let's take a step back and look at the wider picture of why so many of us are struggling.

Chapter 4: Stress, Trauma, and the Gut- Brain Axis

The Emotional Triggers Behind Physical Symptoms

A quick but important note:

While the gut-brain axis plays a powerful role in emotional health, mental health conditions should first be evaluated by a qualified clinician. Traditional mental health care and functional approaches can work together, and the tools in this chapter are intended to support, not replace, professional guidance.

Let's get real: healing your gut isn't just about what's on your plate. I do love a healthy plate, but there's more to it than that. It's also about what's on your mind and in your memory.

We tend to treat stress like background noise. It becomes the soundtrack we live to—the rushing, the pushing, the holding it all together. I know because I lived in that mode for years. I told myself, "This is just life. This is just how I am." But my body had a very different opinion. And it's time to turn that vinyl over!

Chronic stress, old wounds we haven't fully unpacked, emotional overload we keep shoving down...they don't just affect our mood. They change what's happening, physically, inside us. Stress shifts our gut chemistry. It slows digestion, tightens everything up, steals nutrients, and makes it harder for your microbiome to stay balanced. Eventually, all of this shows up as symptoms your doctor might miss entirely.

Bloating, constipation, cravings, rashes, insomnia, hormone swings—these aren't random annoyances. They're messages. They're your body waving a little flag and saying, "Hey, something hurts. Something needs your attention."

This is what survival mode looks like on the inside.

And the moment you stop ignoring those whispers, your healing can finally begin.

Your Gut Has a Nervous System—and It's Listening

By now you've probably figured out your gut is doing a lot more than breaking down dinner. It listens. It reacts. It has a kind of intelligence that most of us never learned to trust. I didn't either, not for a long time.

What shocked me on my healing journey was realizing that my gut actually has its own built-in nervous system—a whole network of nerves sending messages long before my mind could make sense of them. Looking back, my body was speaking to me the whole time. I just didn't know how to hear it yet.

Once you start noticing those signals—the knots, the flutters, the tightness, the sudden cravings, the moments your whole stomach drops—it becomes impossible to ignore how much your gut knows before you do.

My Own Gut-Brain Spiral

Looking back, I noticed a pattern that my worst flare-ups always came during times of unresolved emotional pressure. When I was going through a divorce, my skin flared. When I was building a career, raising kids, and running on coffee and cortisol, my digestion stalled. My candidiasis raged. My body couldn't keep up with the emotional output I was demanding from it.

It wasn't until I discovered meditation and breathwork that I understood how much of my healing would be internal, not just dietary. That first 21-day guided meditation with Deepak Chopra wasn't about silence. It was about returning to myself.

And slowly, my gut followed.

Why This Matters

Once I understood that my gut wasn't reacting in isolation, everything shifted. My symptoms weren't just digestive problems, they were stress problems. Emotional overload, perfectionism, lack of rest, unresolved trauma—all of it was running through my gut first. So, the tools that helped me the most weren't only dietary, they were the ones that calmed my nervous system. When my mind softened, my gut finally had room to heal.

Ways to Support the Gut-Brain Connection

Here's the encouraging part. Once you understand how much your gut and nervous system talk to each other, you can start giving them the support they've been asking for. None of this requires perfection. It's more about coming back to simple, grounding practices that help your body shift out of survival mode and into a state where healing can actually happen. Here are a few things that worked for me:

Breathwork and Meditation: Even a few slow breaths can begin to calm your system. Ten minutes of gentle breathing or quiet meditation signals safety to your body, calming the vagus nerve and helping the gut relax so it can do its job.

Spacious Eating: Giving your body space between meals helps to reset your digestion. When you leave four to five hours between eating, you actually give your body digestive enzymes to sweep your gut clean. If you've been snacking all day (a zone I lived in for years), know that your body is starting another digestive project before finishing the first.

Somatic Practices: Stress doesn't only live in your thoughts. It settles into your tissues. Simple movement practices like stretching, yoga, light shaking, or even standing barefoot on the ground can help release the tension your gut has been holding onto.

Therapeutic Support: If certain stress patterns have followed you for years, you are not weak. You are human. Therapies like EMDR, Internal Family Systems, or other body-focused approaches can help you unwind emotional patterns that keep your gut on edge. Sometimes what your stomach is reacting to isn't food, but feelings that never had a chance to be processed.

The Gut-Brain Axis Is Your Healing Highway

The road to healing isn't just through better probiotics or cutting sugar. Those help, but if you're still running from yourself, your gut never gets the memo that it's safe to restore.

So, here's your invitation: Slow down. Get still. Listen.

Sometimes the most powerful medicine is just...pausing.

Gut Truths to Remember

- Your body isn't betraying you; it's protecting you.
- The gut-brain axis is a two-way street; you can heal from both ends.
- Slowing down isn't a weakness; it's a healing signal.
- If you've "tried everything" but haven't addressed the stress, you haven't tried everything yet.

Once we acknowledge how emotions affect digestion, it becomes clear: food is not just fuel—it's a message.

In the next chapters, we'll decode the messages your meals are sending, and how sugar, processed foods, and inflammation can confuse your body's healing signals.

Coming Up Next

In Chapter 5, we'll finally talk about food—not just *what* to eat, but *why* certain ingredients wreck your gut, and how to build a plate that promotes healing rather than inflammation.

We'll also get into how sugar, processed foods, and the modern diet feed the fungus among us.

Chapter 5: The Role of Diet: Inflammation, Sugar, and Processed Food

How the Modern Plate Fuels the Fungus and Fogs the Mind

You can eat kale and still be bloated. You can be "gluten-free" and still be feeding *Candida*. You can be doing everything right—and still feel wrong.

Why? Because diet isn't just about what's healthy on paper. It's about how food interacts with your gut terrain, hormonal rhythm, and microbial ecosystem. And in a disrupted gut, even "clean" foods can become inflammatory.

Let's break this down. No shame, no diet culture. Just facts, function, and food-as-medicine truth.

Inflammation: The Fire Beneath the Symptoms

At the root of gut dysfunction is often one word: **inflammation—**chronic, silent, systemic, and fueled by what we eat every day. When I was deep in my healing, I would do "just one thing"—remove refined sugar, avoid alcohol, and so on.

Inflammation is a wildfire in the body:

- Triggering gut permeability ("leaky gut")
- Keeping the immune system on high alert
- Disrupting hormonal balance, joint health, and mental clarity
- Allowing *Candida* and "bad bugs" to thrive

And your food is either fighting that fire—or feeding it. We are lucky because we get to choose.

The Sugar–Fungus Connection

Candida albicans is a natural part of your body. It's also smart—and hungry. It looks for sugar to grow.

And it doesn't just live in your gut; it communicates with your brain through the gut-brain axis to trigger sugar cravings. And when you give in to that sugar craving, it thrives and can lead to overgrowth or infections.

Besides feeding *Candida, sugar also*:

- Spikes insulin, which fuels inflammation
- Starves beneficial bacteria, weakening gut defenses
- Crashes mood and energy, driving more cravings
- Ferments in the gut, creating bloating and brain fog

Refined sugar, fruit juices, white flours, and alcohol are all part of the problem.

Even "healthy" sugars like maple syrup, coconut sugar, and honey can be too much when your microbiome is out of balance.

Processed Foods: Empty Calories, Full Damage

Even if you're not eating "fast food," chances are you're still getting processed ingredients in:

- Salad dressings and other condiments
- Protein bars
- "Healthy" crackers and wraps
- Dairy alternatives, loaded with gums, thickeners, or added sugar

These foods:

- Contain industrial seed oils (canola, soybean, safflower), which are prone to oxidation (i.e., breaking down and creating harmful byproducts) and may contribute to inflammation in a body that is sensitive or already inflamed
- Are low in fiber, starving your good gut bacteria
- Often include additives that disrupt digestion

Processed food is designed for **shelf life, not gut life.**

Common "Healthy" Foods That Can Disrupt Healing

Here are some "clean" foods that may be problematic during the gut reset phase:

- **Kombucha**—often high in sugar and yeast
- **Agave nectar**—super high in fructose
- **Cashew yogurt**—can be high in carbs and oxalates
- **Gluten-free breads**—often full of starches and gums
- **Dried fruit**—sugar bomb and high in mold potential
- **Protein bars**—often loaded with sweeteners or fillers

Remember, healing is not about shrinking your world. It's not a forever restriction. It's *temporary precision*, a brief season when your body gets to exhale and repair.

Before I knew that some "healthy" foods were actually problem foods (added sugars, artificial sweeteners, gums), I was making kombucha in my kitchen. I bought all the bottles and fermenting toys. When I learned I was making things worse, with too much caffeine and sugar. I had to reel myself in and say, "*Well, you can't know everything.*" And I learned to let it go.

What to Eat Instead: Healing Foods for a Balanced Gut

Here are some gut-healing "power foods" that worked for me (and what your microbiome is begging for):

Gut-Healing Power Foods

- **Clean proteins:** pasture-raised chicken, wild-caught fish (low-mercury), eggs (if tolerated)
- **Cooked vegetables:** steamed greens, squash, cruciferous veggies
- **Healthy fats:** ghee, olive oil, avocado, nuts and seeds (in moderation)
- **Low-sugar fruits:** kiwi, berries, lemons (in moderation)
- **Fermented foods:** sauerkraut, kimchi, unsweetened coconut yogurt (if tolerated)
- **Prebiotic fibers:** asparagus, onions, garlic, leeks, under-ripe bananas

Pro Tip: Cook or lightly steam (broccoli, cauliflower, kale) during your protocol phase to reduce bloat.

Healing Isn't Just Substitution—It's Transformation

This is not a diet. It's a diagnostic. It's a reset to understand what your body loves and what it resists.

By eliminating inflammatory and fungus-feeding foods, then slowly reintroducing healing ones, you empower your body and your belly to recalibrate.

The bloat subsides. The rash fades. The fog clears. The energy returns.

Your plate becomes a mirror for your microbiome.

What My Functional Medicine Team Recommended

Cynthia Geyer, MD, and nutritionist Annette Quatrano helped me structure my nutrition too:

- Go gluten free, dairy free, and egg free (all the frees!)
- Focus on three meals per day with no snacks to engage the MMC (migrating motor complex)
- Balance plant and animal proteins
- Add calcium citrate to bind oxalates
- Reduce high-oxalate foods (spinach, beets, chocolate, etc.)
- Eat low-mercury fish only (Safe Catch, sardines, salmon)
- Boost protein with vegan powder, collagen, and BCAAs

This wasn't overwhelming, because it was strategic and doable.

Real Gut-Healing Story: Alicia— "The Sugar Crash That Changed Everything"

Alicia, 36, was a busy mom of three with a calendar full of playdates, work calls, and carpool loops. She described herself as a "healthy-ish" eater: smoothies for breakfast, salads when she could, but also a fair share of energy bars, oat milk lattes, and the occasional 3 p.m. cookie just to get through the day.

She thought her sugar cravings were just part of who she was. But when the yeast infections wouldn't stop, the bloating became constant, and she started falling asleep mid-afternoon, she knew something deeper was going on.

After reading about *Candida* and hidden sugar sources, she started the Antifungal protocol from this book—reluctantly cutting even the "natural" sweeteners she thought were harmless.

"The first week was the hardest," she told me. "I was irritable, foggy, and cranky. But by day 10, I woke up clear-headed. That hadn't happened in years."

Now, Alicia starts her mornings with a protein-rich smoothie and preps gut-healing meals on Sundays. She still bakes—just with coconut flour and monk fruit instead of white sugar and flour.

She reflected on the change, saying, "This wasn't a diet. It was a wake-up call. I had no idea how much sugar was ruling my energy, my skin, even my mood."

Your Gut Knows. You Just Forgot How to Listen.

All food isn't the enemy, but it is a message.

And when you start tuning in, you'll realize that your gut has been trying to tell you about it all along.

You don't need another diet. You need a map.

Let's rebuild your plate, your pantry, and your perspective, so your food can finally start healing you instead of hurting you.

Coming Up Next

In Chapter 6, we'll rewrite your nutrition blueprint, including food lists, meal-building strategies, supplement timing, and a plan that works even if you're traveling, working, or managing a busy family.

Healing your gut doesn't require perfection, just alignment.

Chapter 6: Rewriting Your Nutrition Blueprint

Because Your Body Doesn't Want a Diet—It Wants a Map

If food is medicine, then your kitchen is your first pharmacy. But healing doesn't start with restriction—it starts with direction (like you'd give a two-year-old).

You can't nourish a stressed-out body with a stressed-out meal plan. Like going through a drive-through kitchen. It won't end well. And you don't need another crash diet or trendy cleanse, because as soon as those are over, you just restart the madness. You need a blueprint—one that aligns with your symptoms, your lifestyle, and your long-term goals.

This chapter is your invitation to rebuild your nutrition from the inside out—with clarity, confidence, compassion, and yummy food. We'll explore the foods that soothe inflammation, the rhythms that regulate digestion, and the simple principles that turn confusion into clarity.

When I first started healing, even a simple grocery trip felt overwhelming. I stayed on the outside of the store where the real food lived, avoiding the aisles that used to pull me in. I picked out herbs with intention, reading every label (at the beginning) like my life depended on it, because, honestly, it did.

And yes, sometimes I had to wander into the center aisles. But that didn't last long. After a few weeks, the store started to make sense. I knew exactly what my kitchen needed. I knew where the safe ingredients lived. And I stopped feeling like a stranger in my own grocery store.

But I had to start somewhere, and that somewhere was education.

Learning what nourished me.
Learning what harmed me.
Learning how to choose differently.

I remember following “Bobby” on Instagram. He would have different protocols for staying safe in the aisles: buy this, leave that, replace this, add that. I tuned in. I was taking all the advice I could get!

The blueprint begins the same way for you. Not with perfection, but with awareness.

From Elimination to Empowerment

Your gut isn’t skilled only at digestion. It’s also an expert at interpretation. It is constantly scanning for signals of stress or safety, balance or imbalance. That’s why “healthy” food isn’t always healing food.

At the beginning of my journey, I thought I was eating clean: smoothies, kale, salads—check. But my gut was inflamed, my energy unpredictable, and my symptoms persistent.

Here’s what I learned: Healing didn’t come from being stricter. It came from being smarter. It required:

> *Less sugar, more thoughtful replacements*
> *Less guessing, more planning ahead*
> *Less perfection, more purpose*

When I aligned my meals with my gut’s needs (and not just my Pinterest board), everything shifted.

My Detox Jump-Start: The 10-Day Reset That Rewired My Body

Before being accepted into the UltraWellness Center, I took a leap of faith and began Dr. Mark Hyman, MD's "*10-Day Detox.*" Though it was initially designed as a short challenge, it felt so right for my body that I extended it into a full three-month commitment. Intense? Maybe. But it felt like what my body needed, so I listened.

That detox was a turning point because it showed me just how powerful food could be. I was finally reducing inflammation, stabilizing my blood sugar, and clearing my mind. I had energy again. My rashes began to heal. I was becoming my own evidence.

Important Detox Lessons:

- Sugar is not a treat—it's a toxin, especially in a gut that's out of balance.
- Cruciferous veggies, clean proteins, and healthy fats were my main foods.
- Detox doesn't mean deprivation; it means eating with purpose.

What began as a cleanse became a lifelong plan for health.

One thing I might do differently is not go it alone. Community can be a big help to healing.

Your Personalized Nutrition Blueprint Starts Here

This nutrition protocol blends:

- My lived experience with candidiasis, SIBO, IBS, and chronic inflammation
- Results from food sensitivity testing (via Wellevate/Fullscript)

- Expert support from Cynthia Geyer, MD, and nutritionist Annette Quatrano
- Functional medicine principles, including those inspired by Dr. Hyman
- Anti-inflammatory, antifungal, and gut-repair nutritional strategies

Core Goals:

- Starve the fungus, not yourself
- Repair the gut lining
- Reduce systemic inflammation
- Stabilize blood sugar and energy
- Rebuild microbial diversity
- Support hormonal detox and mood balance
- Meal Timing = Motility + Metabolic Healing

Modern snacking habits sabotage a key function: the **Migrating Motor Complex (MMC)**—the internal housekeeping wave of your gut. To activate my MMC and restore my digestive rhythm, I followed Dr. Hyman's structure of three meals a day, spaced four to five hours apart.

This helped to:

- Improve my gut motility
- Reduce fermentation and bloating
- Regulate my blood sugar
- Enhance my parasympathetic ("rest and digest") state

Sample Daily Rhythm:

8:00 AM—Protein-rich breakfast

1:00 PM—Anti-inflammatory, fiber-filled lunch

6:00 PM—Grounding, mineral-rich dinner

Optional—Herbal tea and magnesium at night

The Gut-Healing Plate

Protein (roughly 20–30 g per meal for women, 30–40 g for men)

Wild-caught salmon or sardines
Organic poultry or grass-fed meats
Pasture-raised eggs (if tolerated)
Plant-based proteins (hemp, pea, or rice blends)
Nuts and seeds (check sensitivities)

Cooked Colorful Vegetables

Steamed or roasted cruciferous veggies
Leafy greens: chard, dandelion, bok choy
Roots: carrots, parsnips, squash

Healthy Fats

Avocado
Ghee or coconut oil (antifungal)
Cold-pressed extra-virgin olive oil
Chia, flax, or pumpkin seeds

The idea isn't to restrict for restriction's sake. The goal is to reset your gut terrain, reduce inflammation, and create space for the body to heal.

This isn't punishment, it's freedom in disguise.

Avoid:

Refined sugar and syrups
Fruit juice and dried fruits
White bread, pastries, and cereal
Kombucha (at the beginning)
Starchy carbs that spike blood sugar

Embrace (in moderation):

Low-sugar fruits like berries, grapefruit, and green apples
Herbs such as cinnamon and ginger
Herbal teas—chamomile, dandelion, and fennel

Again, this isn't about lifelong elimination. It's about giving your body what it needs to recover and eventually reintroducing variety with wisdom.

What Actually Worked for Me

Food was my foundation, but supplements, herbs, and targeted support made all the difference. Here's what helped me rebuild trust with my gut:

- Probiotic support (seed, twice daily)
- Sugar-free and fruit-free foods during active *Candida* phase
- Magnesium citrate (AM) + Magnesium Glycinate (PM)
- Motility activator before bed
- Gut food and bitters before meals
- Cooked veggies over raw at the beginning
- Protein with every meal
- BCAAs post-exercise

"Another four weeks to the commitment of the diet. Don't see myself going back..."
— from a personal email after Week 8 of Dr. Hyman's Candida protocol

I relied on traditional medicine for accurate diagnostics, blood work, and oversight, and I paired that medical clarity with functional tools that supported my lifestyle, nervous system, and gut. Both systems informed each step I took.

Coming Up Next

In the next chapter, we'll dive into more of what worked for me—and what may work for you.

Check Out: Your Gut-Safe Grocery Guide

It's time to turn the grocery store into your wellness toolbox. Download the **printable "Gut-Safe Grocery Guide"** at

forwardthinkerwellness.com

Chapter 7: Healing Protocols: Supplements, Herbs & Natural Tools

The Targeted Allies That Brought My Gut Back to Life

You can't out-salad a microbiome crisis. You can't detox stress with just celery juice. And if you've got *Candida* overgrowth, SIBO, or gut inflammation, your body needs reinforcements.

This chapter breaks down the exact supplements, herbal therapies, and natural tools that helped me go from rash-covered, bloated, and exhausted to clear, regular, energized, and deeply well.

This is not a one-size-fits-all supplement list. This is a targeted protocol, built from clinical insight and tested in real life.

First, What Are We Healing?

Before you add another pill to your shelf, know what you're targeting. Most gut-healing journeys, especially for women with stress and hormonal history need to address:

- *Candida* overgrowth (fungal infection from yeast imbalance)
- Bacterial imbalance or SIBO
- Low stomach acid or enzyme insufficiency
- Leaky gut (intestinal permeability)
- Motility dysfunction (constipation)
- Detox overload (mold, mercury, hormone imbalance)
- Nervous-system dysregulation (stress, trauma, imbalance)

Good protocols work in phases, just like functional medicine teaches.

The Three-Phase Protocol

Here's how we built my plan at the UltraWellness Center.

PHASE 1: PREP + PRIMING (Weeks 1–3)

Reduce inflammation, support digestion, calm the system.

Supplements

- **Digestive bitters with turmeric (Gaia Herbs):** Stimulates gastric acid and bile; take 15–20 minutes before meals
- **Magnesium citrate:** 200–400 mg in the morning to support motility
- **Magnesium glycinate:** 200–400 mg at night to support sleep
- **Motility Activator (Integrative Therapeutics):** Ginger + artichoke blend; one capsule twice daily
- **Probiotics (Seed):** Two capsules AM + PM—broad-spectrum, targeted delivery
- Vitamin D + K2 (K-Force): Supports bones and the immune system, and helps keep calcium levels stable after menopause

Lifestyle Tools

- Space meals to 4–5 hours to support "rest and digest."
- Include calming activities like breathwork, walking, or grounding for 10 minutes every day.
- Cut back on or avoid caffeine and alcohol.

PHASE 2: TARGET + TREAT (Weeks 4–10)

Bind, flush, and kill bad fungi and bacteria.

- **Biocidin liquid** (Broad-Spectrum Botanical Blend): Begin with 1 drop three times a day and work your way up to 5 drops three times a day.
- **Berberine** helps keep insulin levels stable and fights *Candida* and bacterial overgrowth.
- **Triphala** is an Ayurvedic herb mix that supports regularity and a gentle detox.
- **Milk thistle** supports the liver during die-off.
- **Evening primrose oil** supports hormone balance, skin, and DGLA (was low in labs).
- **Optional** (depending on labs/symptoms):
  - Calcium citrate 500 mg binds oxalate and protects the kidneys.
  - Collagen peptides help heal connective tissue and the lining of the gut.
  - Activated charcoal helps during flare-ups or when you have been exposed to mold—but don't use with drugs or supplements.

Lifestyle Tools

- Continue spacing your meals.
- Keep workouts moderate (too intense can cause a cortisol spike).
- Do "sweat therapy" once or twice a week in a sauna or through a heated yoga class.

PHASE 3: REINFORCE AND REBUILD (Weeks 11–13 and beyond)

Seal the gut, repopulate good bacteria, restore resilience.

Add or continue:

- **Prebiotic foods (start low + slow):** asparagus, artichokes
- **Gut Food Formula:** probiotic + prebiotic blend

- **Fish oil / Omega-3s:** via supplement or sardines/salmon
- **BCAA powder (Metagenics):** post-workout recovery and protein support
- **DHEA 10 mg (Micronized):** as prescribed; monitor hormones
- **Cortisol Manager:** supports sleep and lowers nighttime cortisol

Lifestyle Tools

- Reintroduce higher-fiber carbs (quinoa, wild rice).
- Let symptoms guide what stays and what is reintroduced later.
- Journal energy, digestion, sleep, and mood daily.

Supplement Timing Snapshot (What and When)

- **Digestive bitters**: 15–20 minutes before meals in a small amount of water to stimulate stomach acid
- **Probiotic (Seed)**: First thing in the morning and again before bed, away from food
- **Motility Activator**: Before breakfast and dinner; avoid taking with binders
- **Magnesium**: Morning and evening for relaxation, motility, and sleep
- **Biocidin**: Between meals; begin low and build slowly to minimize die-off
- **Berberine / milk thistle**: With meals to protect gut and liver while balancing blood sugar
- **BCAAs**: Before or during workouts for muscle recovery
- **Cortisol Manager**: 30–60 minutes before bed to support restful sleep
- **DHEA**: In the morning, in low doses, under professional guidance

Real Talk: You Don't Need 50 Pills a Day

I remember those early days so clearly. My kitchen counter was covered with teas, supplements, sticky notes, and labels. I had lists for everything. It was organized chaos, and, yes, it felt like a lot. But I also learned something important along the way: most of it was temporary.

This protocol may look complex, but it's simpler than most. The secret is sequencing, knowing what your body needs right now and what can wait. And just like I did, you'll taper off several of these once the acute phase passes. Supplements are there to support a season of healing, not to replace your body's wisdom forever. Just breathe and hang in there!

My Healing Timeline: What I Felt, When

Weeks 2–3: Daily bowel movements returned, and my energy stayed stable by midday.

Weeks 4–5: *Candida* rash faded, and bloating after meals decreased.

Weeks 6–7: Sleep deepened, and sugar cravings dropped dramatically.

Weeks 8–10: Brain fog lifted, skin cleared, and mood steadied.

Week 11 and beyond: Workout energy increased, and confidence in food rhythm rose.

You're Not Alone, You're Not Broken

Feeling overwhelmed, so many protocols to keep track of. What to eat, what not to eat, which supplements, at what time. This is the moment in healing where many give up or lose heart.

If your skin flares, your bowels slow, or your cravings return, just pause. Adjust. Breathe. Don't panic.

You are rebalancing.

Coming Up Next

In Chapter 8, we'll get physical, exploring the movement, breathwork, and somatic rituals that support healing of the gut and nervous system. We'll talk about how I used breathwork and bodywork to bring life back to my tissues and stillness back to my nervous system.

You've got this!

Chapter 8: My Gut-Body Healing Routine

Gut Healing Requires Safety, Not Just Strategy

> "Trust the body. It was built to heal when given the right signals."

You can eat all the right things, take every supplement on time, and still feel off, bloated, anxious, and stuck, because your body isn't in a healing state.

Why? Because your nervous system hasn't gotten the signal that it's safe. Once internal healing begins, the body naturally asks for movement—gentle, intentional, and restorative.

When your body feels safe enough to rest, break down, and absorb nutrients, good digestion happens, and you can thrive!

And most of us? We're eating while:

- Scrolling
- Driving
- Watching the news
- Stressing about our to-do list
- Running on adrenaline

This slows down:

- Gastric acid production
- Enzyme secretion
- Motility
- Gut blood flow

Self-Care: The Simplest Gut-Healing Tool on Earth

A huge part of my reset came through my dedication to Kripalu, the beautiful yoga retreat center in the Berkshires. I found peace and power on the mat and was endlessly inspired by longtime yogi Jurian Hughes, whose joyful energy made me think, "I want to feel that free again."

Her yoga dance and bodywork teachings, especially during a retreat in Mexico, offered me a safe space to soften, listen, and reconnect. The retreat sat between the ocean and the jungle, where mornings began with sunlight spilling over the horizon and evenings ended with laughter, reflection, and the sound of waves.

We practiced in open-air studios, with warm breezes, the sound of birds, and the smell of ocean water. We were barefoot on warm tile. Jurian's classes combined dance, movement, and meditation in a combination that seemed both ancient and fresh.

Her presence was radiant—joyful yet deeply grounded—inviting us to move from our truth, not our tension. With her gentle guidance, I was able to let go and heal without having to work at it. I kept practicing with Jurian through her online lessons after I returned from the retreat. Her energy came through the screen just as brightly as it did in person. Those virtual sessions helped me keep on track between trips by reminding me to breathe deeply, move slowly, and reconnect with myself even on busy days.

I also found grounding through somatic journaling and movement workshops with Jess Frey, the Lead Faculty at Kripalu. Her steady presence and contemplative practices helped me throughout the quieter seasons of my healing. Her work offered me a soft landing, especially on days when my nervous system needed more tenderness than structure.

It wasn't just yoga. It was a remembrance, a homecoming to my body, to safety, and to peace.

Advance Praise

"Jackie's journey is a powerful reminder that healing happens through presence, courage, and deep listening. This book weaves science, story, and spirit in a way that invites real transformation. A beautiful companion for anyone ready to reclaim their vitality."
—Jurian Hughes, Senior Faculty, Kripalu School of Yoga; E-RYT 500, YACEP

One of the most powerful turning points in my healing came not through supplements or food, but through movement. Not fitness, not force, but embodied, intuitive movement that helped me feel again.

Consistent massage therapy was also key. It wasn't just relaxation—it was a way to physically release stored tension and inflammation from my body.

Movement and Breathwork for Healing

If food is fuel and supplements are tools, then movement is the ignition. And breath? Breath is the language your nervous system understands best.

Your vagus nerve is the main messenger between your gut and brain. It tells your digestive system when to slow down or speed up, depending on whether you're safe.

Breath is the on-switch for the vagus nerve.

The following is something I do while I wait at red lights... Try it:

Take a deep breath right now, in through your nose for 4 counts, hold for 2, out through your mouth for 6.

That longer exhale? It literally shifts your body into rest-and-digest mode.

Through this process I learned just 10 minutes of daily breathwork can:

- Reduce cortisol
- Lower blood pressure
- Improve gut motility
- Decrease symptoms of IBS and anxiety
- Increase microbial diversity (via vagus-nerve stimulation)

Real Gut-Healing Story: Lena— "Body Anxious, Breath Calm"

Lena, who was 29, had been dealing with anxiety for more than ten years. For a while, meditation apps helped. Prescribed drugs made her symptoms less severe, but they never made her feel whole.

She didn't really feel in her body. Her breathing was shallow. Her shoulders were constantly at her ears.

That changed when she learned about how to regulate her nervous system and repair her own body. It wasn't just about mindset—it was about motion.

She started walking slowly every morning, without her phone (well played). Then came the time for some breathwork: 4-7-8 breathing before bed. Then there was yin yoga. And a few other suggestions. As she went, Lena said, "I realized I didn't need to work out harder. I needed to feel safe in my body."

Lena's digestion improved. Her panic attacks became rare. And for the first time in years, she said, "I feel like I'm home in my skin."

For me, everything changed when I stopped chasing control and started building flow.

Breathwork taught me how to regulate, not override.

Movement taught me how to release, not hold on for dear life.

And slowly, my gut responded.

Gut-Loving Movement: What to Do (and What to Stop Doing)

Healing-Friendly Movement:

- Walking (especially post-meal): 10–20 minutes improves motility and blood sugar.
- Gentle yoga or stretching
- Rebounding (mini-trampoline)
- Strength training (E-Gym or body weight)
- Dancing: Joy moves the gut!

Gut-Disruptive Movement:

- Overtraining (sounds good at the time)
- Workouts while fasting and under-slept (overstresses the body)
- Workouts that leave you drained instead of energized (seems obvious but wasn't always for me)

Listen to your nervous system. If your workout mimics a stress response, your gut won't thank you.

Breath is free and transformative. Trust in the process! Here are three five-minute daily breath rituals you can try:

- Box Breathing: inhale through your nose, hold, exhale, and hold again for the same number of seconds.

- 4-7-8 Breathing: inhale through your nose for four seconds, hold your breath for seven seconds, exhale slowly out your mouth for eight seconds.
- Alternate Nostril Breathing: breathe through one nostril while holding the other with your fingers closed, switch and exhale through the other.

I remember years ago during my healing journey, shortly after I started deep meditation. I got home from work and put my keys and phone in a dish in the kitchen and didn't touch them for the entire weekend. I stayed within myself and was in and out of meditation for the entire weekend. Believe me when I say, it was one of the best weekends of my life. There is such power when you can hold yourself and know your higher power won't let you down.

Gut Truths to Move With:

Stillness is medicine.
Rest is productive.
Gentle is powerful.

Coming Up Next

In chapter 9, we'll redefine detox—not as punishment, but as a profound return to clarity and self-respect. It's not just what you remove. It's how you support what stays.

Chapter 9: Detoxing from Stress, Toxins, and Emotional Blocks

Detox Without Deprivation

Some people detox with green juices. Others need to detox from pressure, people-pleasing, mold exposure, and childhood survival patterns. *Because healing isn't just about what you remove, it's about what you restore.* Your gut can't heal in a body that feels unsafe—or in a world full of unfiltered toxins.

Environmental Load: Mold, Mercury, and More

I once stayed in a cottage in Maine. It looked charming...until I found black mold on the walls. My body reacted with fatigue, headache, sore throat, and congestion. Mold, heavy metals like mercury, and chemical exposures aren't minor concerns. They're silent triggers of inflammation—and they disrupt the gut and brain profoundly. I'll talk about my mold experience (and how to deal with mold) in more detail in chapter 14.

Detox Upgrade That Changed Everything

After learning how toxins accumulate, I made one of my most impactful upgrades: I invested in the **AquaTru Water System**—also recommended by Dr. Hyman and featured at *forwardthinkerwellness.com*.

It's NSF-certified and removes:

- Fluoride
- PFAs ("forever chemicals")
- Arsenic
- Hormone disruptors
- Pesticides

Your detox doesn't need to start with a cleanse—it can start with clean water.

Toxin Awareness + DIY Shift

One day I had a realization: the toxins were everywhere. If I couldn't control everything, I could at least control what I put on and around my body. I started making my own body lotions, deodorant, toothpaste, household cleaners, laundry detergent, and scrubs—some of which I gifted to friends, family, and clients.

I'm not perfect. I'm just trying. And that alone is powerful.

DIY Environmental Detox

Real wellness happens in your kitchen...and in your cleaning cabinet. You can't detox your body if your physical environment keeps re-toxifying it. The good news? You can clean up your space—without toxic chemicals.

Jackie's Quick-Swaps

Bathroom

- Replace fragranced dryer sheets with wool balls. Add a few drops of essential oils to each ball for a natural scent.
- Trade conventional toothpaste for DIY versions made with coconut oil and baking soda.
- For body odor, try magnesium oil spray, a natural deodorant, or your own recipe!

Kitchen

- Swap plastic containers for glass storage.
- Use vinegar and citrus for surface cleaning.
- Choose cast iron, stainless steel, or ceramic cookware over synthetic non-stick pans like Teflon.

Cleaning Cabinet

- Ditch bleach-based sprays for essential-oil blends.
- Add a blend of purifying essential oils (clove, lemon, cinnamon, eucalyptus, and rosemary) to homemade soap.
- Make a natural cleaning spray with essential oils: Mix 1 cup water + 1 cup vinegar + 10 drops lavender + 10 drops lemon in a glass spray bottle.

DIY Detox Blends Using Essential Oils

- **Calm + Clean Air Spray:** lavender, eucalyptus, tea tree, or lemon
- **Liver Love Roll-On:** castor-oil base + rosemary + peppermint
- **Foot Spray:** magnesium chloride + lavender + frankincense (great before bed!)

Tip from the road: My lavender-oil eye mask is a nervous-system saver on planes. Don't forget to bring your DIY detox toolkit when traveling!

Recipes for Clean Cleaning

When I started to understand how many chemicals were hiding in everyday products—toothpaste, deodorant, dish soap, even laundry detergent—I realized my body couldn't fully heal in a toxic environment.

So I took matters into my own hands. Literally.

At first, it was about control—doing what I could with what I had. But it quickly became about joy. I was crafting little jars of self-respect. I was reclaiming my environment. I was turning my home into a healing sanctuary.

Some of these became daily staples. Others I gave as gifts to friends and family. And the best part? People kept asking for more.

Homemade Toothpaste

A clean mouth shouldn't come with a side of parabens or artificial sweeteners.

Ingredients:

- 3 tbsp coconut oil
- 1½ tbsp baking soda
- 10 drops peppermint essential oil
- 5 drops tea tree oil (optional)

Directions: Mix into a smooth paste and store in a small glass jar. Use a clean wooden spatula or spoon to scoop (no double-dipping).

Detox Body Scrub

This one smells like a spa—and works like one too.

Ingredients:

- ½ cup organic cane sugar or fine Himalayan salt
- ¼ cup coconut oil or olive oil
- Zest of 1 lemon or a few drops of your favorite essential oil

Directions: Combine, store in a glass jar, and use 1–2×/week on damp skin. Rinse well.

Natural Deodorant

Yes, it actually works—and no, it won't leave you smelling like earthy (unless you want to).

Ingredients:

- 3 tbsp Shea butter
- 3 tbsp coconut oil
- ¼ cup arrowroot powder
- 2 tbsp baking soda (reduce if sensitive)
- 10 drops lavender or tea tree essential oil

Directions: Melt oils, stir in powders and essential oils, pour into a tin or tube, and let set. Apply with clean fingers or spoon.

All-Purpose Citrus Cleaner

A spray that sparkles—without ammonia, bleach, or synthetic fragrance. Sounds like a commercial. But I am not selling it, yet!

Ingredients:

- Peels from two to three lemons or oranges
- 1 cup white vinegar
- 1 cup filtered water
- 10 drops lemon or lavender essential oil

Directions: Soak peels in vinegar for 1–2 weeks. Strain and combine with water and essential oils in a spray bottle.

DIY Laundry Soap

No sulfates or mystery chemicals—just clean, soft clothes.

Ingredients:

- 1 bar of unscented castile soap, grated
- 1 cup washing soda
- 1 cup baking soda
- Optional: a few drops of lavender or eucalyptus oil

Directions: Mix and store with a scoop. Use 2–3 tbsp per load.

Tip: Use the above directions precisely, my first couple batches left me a bit spotty... It was a bit of live and learn, play, and figure it out.

Simple Dish Soap

Gentle enough for hands, strong enough for grease.

Ingredients:

- 1 cup unscented castile soap
- 1 tbsp baking soda
- 10 drops lemon or tea tree oil

Directions: Mix in a squeeze bottle. Shake before each use.

Emotional Load: Invisible Toxicity

You can't lab-test your emotional load. You can't track it in grams. But stress is real—and it inflames everything.

Divorce, career shifts, people-pleasing.
Loss, betrayal, burnout.
Childhood trauma or emotional neglect.
Over-giving and under-receiving.

All of this registers in the body. The gut hears it all. You're not "too sensitive"—your body is responding intelligently.

Detoxing Emotionally (Without Losing Yourself)

I've spent years letting go of physical toxins—and just as long clearing the emotional ones. Through breathwork, Reiki, somatic movement, and journaling, I created a rhythm of release without breakdown.

Here's what I learned:

- You don't need to re-live trauma to release it.

- Crying is a detox, literally.
- Saying “no” is a form of liver support.
- Grounding is better than ghosting.
- Gratitude lowers cortisol.

“Toxic Positivity” Is Still Toxic

You don’t have to feel grateful for illness, betrayal, or loss. But you can honor how your body survived it. No one should have to smile through suffering or seem like a hard time was “meant to be.” It’s not about ignoring what happened as you heal. It’s about being thankful that your body got you through times when you weren’t sure it would make it.

Being truly grateful doesn’t mean being grateful for the bad times. It’s about seeing how strong you are, how your nervous system adapted, how you kept fighting, and how you didn’t give up.

How to Support Lymphatic Flow—Your Detox Highway

Your lymphatic system is like the trash-removal crew of your body, the lymphatic fluid helping to carry away toxins, waste, and pathogens. But unlike your heart, the lymphatic system doesn’t pump on its own. It relies on movement, breath, and hydration.

Daily Lymphatic Support Checklist

- **Dry Brushing:** Before your shower, use a natural bristle brush and sweep toward your heart.
- **Rebounding:** A mini-trampoline isn’t just fun—it’s one of the best ways to stimulate lymph. Even five minutes counts.
- **Contrast Showers:** Alternate hot and cold water to boost circulation and drainage. End on cold for an energizing finish.

- **Hydration + Lemon:** Lymph is mostly water. Add a pinch of sea salt or fresh lemon to your drinking water for mineral support.
- **Movement:** Walking, yoga, or dancing—anything that gets you moving helps move lymph too.

Real Gut-Healing Story: Mark—"From Burnout to Balance"

Mark, 42, had a full life—and a depleted body. His fast-paced job in tech, two young kids, and back-to-back meetings left him wired but tired. His skin broke out with psoriasis. His brain fog was so thick, he'd re-read the same email three times.

He blamed stress. He blamed aging. He blamed genetics. It wasn't until he read about the gut-emotion-toxicant connection that something clicked.

He stopped saying yes to every project and every invitation. He tossed the synthetic air fresheners and swapped his cleaning products. He added journaling and daily walks—just 15 minutes after work. He also started tracking his symptoms and logging food, sleep, mood, and flare-ups.

> "The biggest detox I did wasn't with charcoal. It was with boundaries."

His psoriasis faded. His digestion steadied. And he learned how to spot stress before it took him down.

My Daily Gut Reset Journal

Healing your gut isn't just about what you eat. It's *about* what you think, feel, and believe. This journal is your daily invitation to slow down, listen, and partner with your body.

You can start any day of the week.

Use the template below as your sample daily self-guide and explore the companion *From Soil to Soul: Rooted & Renewed™ Daily Reset Journal & Devotional* for the full 90-day journey with expanded reflection pages, affirmations and healing prompts.

Daily Gut Reset Template

Date:

Sleep / Energy / Mood:

Meals & Supplements:

Movement / Hydration:

Gut Tracker: (Bloating | Cravings | BM | Skin | Stress)

Wins or Shifts:

Today's Affirmation:

Gratitude:

Reflection / Prayer / Note to Self:

Healing is often Sadness before it shines.

Gut-Mind Reflection Prompts: Daily & Weekly Journaling for Emotional Detox and Gut Healing

To help you embody this lifestyle shift, use the following prompts as gentle invitations inward. These questions aren't meant to fix you—they're meant to reconnect you to the wisdom already inside you.

Try choosing one or two per day, or use them as weekly check-ins.

Emotional Detox + Nervous System Support

- What have I been holding in—emotionally or physically?
- Where in my life am I over-giving and under-receiving?
- What's something I can let go of today that no longer aligns?
- What loving boundary can I honor this week?
- What does safety feel like in my body—and how can I return to it?

Gut-Brain Communication

- What symptom showed up today—and what might it be trying to say?
- If my gut had a voice, what would it be asking for?
- Did I nourish my body today or just feed it?
- What emotion might be living in my digestive system right now?

Grief, Gratitude, and Growth

- Which part of me is healing—even if it doesn't look like it yet?
- What are three things my body has done for me today?
- What am I still grieving—and how can I hold space for that?
- Which part of my healing journey am I proud of?

Vision & Integration

- What does wellness look like for the future version of me?
- What habits am I cultivating that my future self will thank me for?
- What would healing feel like in my relationships, not just my body?
- If I fully believed I could heal, what would I do differently this week?

The Bigger Picture

Each of these small shifts became ceremonies in my healing. They reminded me: I'm not just detoxing my body—I'm detoxing my life.

Clean living is not about fear, and it is not about perfection. It's about trying your best and letting the rest go. I remind myself of this each day.

You don't have to do everything at once. Start with one. See how it feels. Eventually it will become second nature.

> *You don't have to respond flawlessly. You just have to show up or slow down whatever is going on with you in this moment. Your gut will do the rest.*

Coming Up Next

In chapter 10, we'll put it all together—bringing your gut healing into your real, messy, beautiful life.

Healing isn't a diet. It's a lifestyle.

Chapter 10: Rebuilding the Gut-Brain Axis

Advanced Insights into the Microbiome, Vagus Nerve & Emotional Release

Your gut is more than just a machine for digesting food; it's your second brain.

Your gut has more than 100 million neurons and trillions of bacteria, so it doesn't just respond to your brain; it talks back. In fact, 90% of the messages that go between your gut and your brain flow upward—from your belly to your thoughts. Yes, *gut to the brain*.

When this axis is disrupted, through stress, trauma, infections, or poor diet, you don't just feel bloated. You feel anxious, disconnected, depressed, tired, and triggered.

The good news is you can rebuild it.

This chapter talks about the most advanced, research-backed tools that can help you repair the link between your gut and brain and start real, sustainable healing from the inside out.

Microbiome = Mood Engine

Your microbes are little chemical factories. They make more than 30 distinct neurotransmitters, such as serotonin, dopamine, and GABA, which have a direct effect on your mood, sleep, focus, and ability to bounce back.

An imbalanced gut can cause neuroinflammation, leaky gut, leaky brain, and mood swings.

The Vagus Nerve: Your Healing Superhighway

The vagus nerve is the main route connecting your gut and your brain.

When it is toned and working well, it helps with digestion, keeps inflammation in check, keeps your heart rate and breathing steady, and makes you feel peaceful, safe, and connected to others.

When it isn't working right, digestion slows down, anxiety goes up, and healing stalls.

Tools to Stimulate the Vagus Nerve

You do not need a prescription—you need practice. The tools that follow are ones you can practice to aid your healing journey.

Acupuncture: An ancient Chinese treatment that uses small needles to release chemicals that help with pain and make you feel better. *This was one of the most transformative tools that helped my nervous system work better. The mix of breathing, needles, and deep relaxation brought my body from survival mode to safety. I could sense right away that acupuncture helped release stored tension, decrease inflammation, and encourage whole-body healing.*

Breathwork and meditation, especially breathing from the diaphragm: Deep, slow breathing wakes up the parasympathetic nervous system and increases vagus nerve activity.

Singing loudly or gargling: These stimulate the vagal motor fibers in your throat. *Singing in your car or at church is a form of gut therapy!*

Cold exposure (shower or face splash): A quick cold shower or putting cold water on your face works your blood vessels and vagus nerve. *Not my personal favorite, but hey, "no pain, no gain."*

Humming, chanting, or OM-ing: The sound of your voice and chest vibrating stimulates the vagal branches and soothes the nervous system.

Letting Go of Emotions: The Gut Remembers

Trauma isn't merely something that happens in your mind. It leaves an imprint within your body, especially in your gut. During my healing, I practiced letting go in these ways:

Body-Based Practices: Yoga, massage therapy, and even dancing (*alone in my kitchen!*) released tension stored in and around my muscles.

Journaling + Emotional Release: Putting words to my experience helped move stuck emotions, especially grief.

Community and Conversation: Being witnessed in my healing journey was more powerful than any probiotic. I have said it a thousand times*: we are meant to live in communion, not silos.*

Faith: Leaning into belief in something greater than myself gave me resilience and spiritual steadiness.

Bringing Together the Mind and the Soul

Your biology and biography are not two different things; they are one. You're not just changing what you eat; you're also rewriting the story your body tells itself. *Your gut is listening.*

Be curious about how your nervous system works. Ask yourself:

When do I feel safe in my body?
When do I tighten or contract without realizing it?
Which meals make me feel better?

You are amazing! Know it, feel it, live it, eat it. Pour into yourself and your health. Be your own best friend! You're worth it.

The Divine Appointment

There was a day in my healing journey that felt less like coincidence and more like guidance. I remember walking barefoot in the park, on the phone, talking with my sister, and crying because I was not well. My mind was overwhelmed, my gut was inflamed, and my nervous system was spiraling. I felt lost in my own body.

I decided to push through the chaos and find an acupuncturist. I needed to do *something*. I tried two different places that afternoon, hoping for help. The first was closed. The second was not open yet. Every door felt shut.

By the grace of God and the internet I found George.

I texted him on instinct, hoping for an appointment. He thought I was already an existing client, so he stuck to the appointment, even though he was not taking new clients at the time. Somehow, through what felt like a small crack in the universe, he told me to come in.

When I walked through his door, everything shifted. He listened. He pulled me into the present. He helped my nervous system settle enough for my body to even consider healing. Then he began a whole-body treatment that reached places nothing else had touched. It felt like something in me finally exhaled, like my system remembered what safety felt like. It changed me from the inside out.

It was more than luck. It was a divine appointment, the moment my body felt safe enough to take the next step.

Coming Up Next

You have learned how to rebalance, reboot, and rebuild. In the next chapter, we'll talk about staying well, even when life gets messy or hectic.

Because *maintenance* is the real magic. You've got this!

Chapter 11: Regulation + Emotional Triggers

Fight, Flight, Freeze, and Flare

It's one of the most overlooked truths in wellness: you can be doing everything right—perfect supplements, flawless foods, all the right labs—but if your nervous system is stuck in survival mode, your gut won't get the memo to relax, digest, and repair.

You can't gut-heal your way out of a fight-or-flight life.

If you grew up in a home where stress was constant, boundaries were blurred, or you had to stay small to stay safe, your nervous system adapted. But wiring for survival isn't the same as wiring for wellness.

You might:

- Wake up anxious for no reason
- Freeze or feel fearful when conflict arises
- People-please or overwork to earn safety
- Feel exhausted after social interaction

These aren't defects in your character. But you can change them by rewriting them.

Awareness of Triggers = Power

A trigger isn't the problem. It's our unconscious reaction to it that requires our efforts.

To regain power over these triggers:

- Identify the people, places, or patterns that tend to dysregulate you.
- Build micro-boundaries that protect your energy.

- Rehearse a safe response in your mind before real moments arise (respond vs. react).

"Regulation isn't perfection. It's choosing safety one moment at a time."

Real Gut-Healing Story: Daniel— "Finding Calm in a Fight-or-Flight World"

Daniel, 35, was the last guy you'd expect to embrace cold showers and vagus-nerve exercises. He ran a digital agency, drank espresso like water, and thought meditation was for monks.

After three months of stomach pain, insomnia, and a tight chest, he hit pause.

At first, it was breathwork before bed. Then cold exposure. Then humming in the shower (which he swore he'd never admit to doing, until it worked).

His digestion improved. His heart-rate variability increased. He felt calmer and clearer. He reflected later, "I didn't need a new diet. I needed a new pace."

Daniel still works hard, but now he:

- Eats lunch mindfully without screens
- Does three minutes of deep breathing before meetings, and at red lights
- Sleeps better than he has in years

A Day in the Life of a Gut-Healing Traveler: Living Well, Even on the Go

Travel is rarely predictable. Delayed flights, missed trains, and rushed transitions can throw anyone off. But when you're on a gut-healing journey, those small interruptions can feel massive. Preparation isn't just helpful—it's essential.

On a whirlwind trip to Europe, I learned the value of thinking ahead—scouring menus for gut-friendly options, stopping at farm stands, and politely requesting olive oil and lemon at bistros.

One favorite strategy? Making my own snacks before chaos begins. During a mad dash to catch a train to New York City, I relied on my trusted travel kit:

- Homemade protein balls with coconut oil, flaxseed, and sprouted granola
- Avocado ("nature's butter")
- Lemons for travel hydration
- Purified water bottle with built-in filter
- Chopped figs rolled in coconut flakes—a nourishing, sweet alternative
- Mini pouch with herbal teas, supplements, and digestive enzymes

In the city, I even found a natural health-food store nearby—proof that where there's a will, there's a way to stay well.

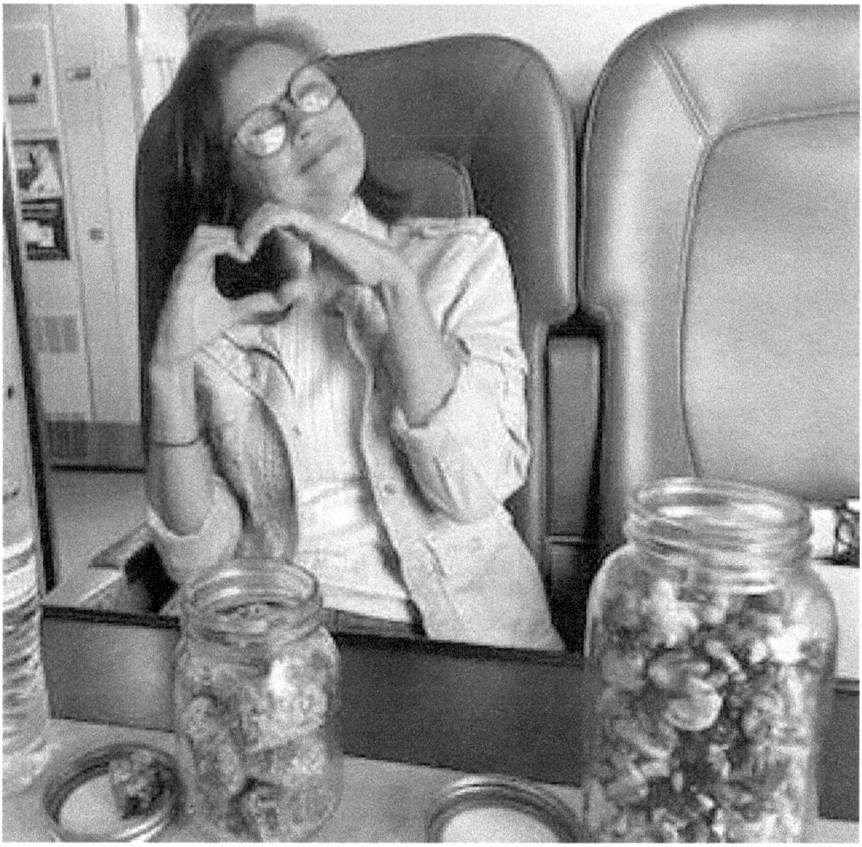

Travel essentials: homemade snacks, nuts, gratitude, peace, laughter and friends. Thank you -GM!

The Gut-Healing Carry-On Checklist

- Reusable water bottle with filter
- Small container of Celtic sea salt and lemon for morning hydration
- Protein balls, nuts, seeds, olive packs, or low-sugar fruit
- Travel-size olive oil and coconut oil for meals
- Herbal teas: chamomile, ginger, peppermint, pau d'Arco
- Activated charcoal (for food mishaps)

- Bitters or enzymes for meals out
- Eye mask and magnesium or a calming spray for sleep
- Lavender oil, small journal, and blue-light glasses for nervous-system care
- A list of two or three “safe” restaurants or a natural market in advance
- Breathwork + stretches in the hotel room or airport lounge

You don’t need to be perfect, just prepared. When your body feels safe, supported, and nourished, healing becomes a lifestyle, not a location.

Coming Up Next

You’ve worked on food. You’ve cleaned your space. In chapter 12, you’ll learn how to listen deeper, to the emotional undercurrents that have been shaping your gut’s resilience.

Chapter 12: Holistic Lifestyle Integration

Where Gut Healing and Prayer Become a Way of Life

You've tracked your meals, taken the supplements, changed your breakfast, and learned about prebiotics and probiotics. *But healing doesn't end when your protocol does.*

It evolves.

It's not a diet; it's a way of life that includes making everyday choices that help your mind, body, and gut work together. And that way of life involves both standard and alternative medicine. If you need medical help, medication, tests, or advice, that's all part of your healing. Functional medicine is just a way to help you fix what standard medicine finds.

I started to identify a trend based on both study and my own life. People who really healed their gut and kept it that way didn't simply change what they ate; they also changed how they lived. Over time, I started to put this together into what I call **"The Five Pillars of a Gut-Healing Lifestyle"**:

1. **Food as Fuel (and Feedback)**: You're not dieting, you're dialoguing with your body. Ask yourself: Did that meal give me more energy or make me feel worse?
2. **Restorative Movement**: Not to burn calories, but to move toxins, support digestion and motility, and calm the nervous system. (Think of going for walks, doing yoga, going to the gym, or lifting weights.)
3. **Ritualized Rest**: Sleep isn't a luxury; it's therapy for your gut. Cortisol drops, cells are repaired, and inflammation resets. Relax and wind down with magnesium glycinate, herbal tea, and a digital sunset.

4. **Community + Joy**: Connection heals. Whether it's having dinner with friends, coaching others, or playing Mexican Train, these are the anti-inflammatory nutrients we often forget about. People need connection.
5. **Spiritual + Emotional Reset**: Prayer, reiki, meditation, breathwork, or simply sitting in nature all teach your body one message: You are safe now.

A Day in the Life: Example Routines for Healing

The following routines are examples for helping people heal in the midst of their own challenging lifestyles.

The Busy Working Mom

Meet Jen, 42, mom of two, juggling work, kids' schedules, and her own healing from candidiasis and fatigue. She needs structure but flexibility.

Morning (6:30 AM)

Wake-Up Ritual: Gratitude list (3 things), lemon water with sea salt

Breakfast (7:15 AM):

- Scrambled pasture-raised eggs with sauteed spinach and mushrooms in ghee
- Half an avocado
- Herbal tea with ginger and cinnamon
- Supplements: Probiotic (seed), magnesium citrate, digestive enzyme (if needed)

Midday

Quick Break (11:00 AM): 10-minute breathwork or walk outside

Lunch (12:30 PM):

Digestive bitters before meal
Baked salmon with steamed broccoli and roasted carrots
Quinoa with olive oil

Mindset Check-In: “How do I feel emotionally right now?”

Evening (6:30 PM)

Dinner:

Ground turkey sauteed with zucchini and garlic
Cauliflower mash
Herbal tea (peppermint or chamomile)

Kids’ Bedtime (8:30 PM): They journal, so she journals too.

Self-Care: Epsom salt bath and one capsule Motility Activator

Lights Out: 9:30 PM with phone on airplane mode

Why It Works

- Predictable meal timing supports motility.
- Cooked veggies improve digestion.
- Tiny mindset and breath break lower cortisol and enhance gut flow.

The Burned-Out Entrepreneur

Meet Alex, 35, self-employed, used to skipping meals and living on caffeine. He has finally committed to healing from brain fog, bloating, and burnout.

Morning (7:30 AM)

Wake-Up Ritual: 5-minute vagus nerve activation (deep humming and breathwork)

Breakfast (8:15 AM):

Protein smoothie with pea protein, chia, frozen zucchini, cinnamon, and almond milk
1 hard-boiled egg
Supplements: Magnesium and L-Glutamine

Midday

Lunch (1:00 PM):

Digestive bitters before eating
Salad with arugula, grilled chicken, roasted beets, pumpkin seeds, and olive oil
Small serving of sweet potato

3:00 PM: 10-minute power nap or Muse meditation session

Evening (6:30 PM)

Dinner:

Brothy soup with lentils, carrots, and dandelion greens
1 slice cassava flatbread with avocado
Herbal tea (dandelion root)

Night Stack: Probiotic, glycinate, B-complex, Motility Activator

Wind-Down: 10 pages of spiritual reading

Sleep: 10:00 PM sharp with blackout curtains and Oura ring tracking

Why It Works

- No grazing stabilizes glucose and energy.
- Strategic supplements support brain and gut.
- Spiritual time rewires stress pathways.

The Recovering Perfectionist

Maria, 39, well versed in "clean eating" and overachieving. Now she is recovering from orthorexia, SIBO, and anxiety. She is learning how to be flexible, trust her gut, and be kind to herself.

Morning (7:00 AM)

Wake-Up: No screens. Sit in stillness for two minutes.

Breakfast (7:45 AM):

- Warming porridge of cauliflower rice, hemp milk, cinnamon, and chia
- Scrambled egg on the side

Mantra: "Slow is healing. Soft is strong."

Midday

Lunch (1:00 PM):

- Stir-fry with ground lamb, bok choy, carrots, and coconut aminos
- Small portion of white rice—no more fear!

Mid-Afternoon Practice: Emotional Freedom Technique (EFT tapping)

Snack (if needed): Handful of walnuts with tea

Evening (6:45 PM)

Dinner:

- Apple cider vinegar before eating
- Baked cod, steamed kale, mashed parsnips

Reflection: "What did I trust today?"

Magnesium and bedtime prayer

Why It Works

- Honors the nervous system over tracking macronutrients and calories.
- Transforms perfectionism into being present.
- Blends emotional tools with food freedom.

Your Gut-Life Alignment List

This is something you could try every Sunday to get your week off to a good start:

- Did I plan some movement that feels good?
- Did I make at least three meals that are healthy for my gut?
- Do I have time set aside for sufficient sleep, breathwork, and journaling?
- What is one thing I'm planning to do that will bring me joy?
- What help do I need this week?

A Note on Spirit and Source

Food and exercise helped my body heal, but faith kept my spirit strong.

That deeper connection—whether you call it God, source, the universe, or anything else—gave me the fortitude to keep going. On the hardest days, when the rash came back or I thought I would never get well, I turned to prayer, presence, and the belief that something bigger than me was helping me through.

Healing is sacred work. Trusting that I wasn't alone, even when I felt isolated, and leaning into the power of prayer, He helped me rebuild not just my gut, but my resilience too.

So wherever you are on your journey, connect with that still place within. That quiet, sacred voice that whispers, "Don't give up yet." I believe in you!

When you start to feel better, a new question comes up: How do I stay better?

Coming Up Next

Your goal is no longer to heal your gut; it's your foundation. In the next chapter, we'll talk about what it means to live in prevention rather than reaction, and you'll learn how to protect your progress and do well even after the symptoms go away.

Chapter 13: The Preventative Mindset for Lifelong Gut-Brain Health

Preventative Mindset for Lifelong Health

For most of us, "normal" has meant:

- Pushing through stress
- Skipping meals or snacking all day
- Eating foods, we knew didn't serve us
- Blaming aging, hormones, or genetics
- Thinking "this is just the way I am"

You've now proven otherwise.

Getting better, however, isn't the end. It's the beginning of a new way of living. By the time you get to this chapter, you've likely begun to experience what's possible: clearer skin, better digestion, fewer energy crashes, less brain fog, fewer rashes, and more joy.

But I have to be honest with you: healing your gut isn't something you can just check off and forget about. It's constant planning, making the right choices for your body, keeping your energy up, keeping your gut happy, and maintaining a deep relationship with your inner self. And like all relationships, it requires ongoing attention, trust, and care.

Visual Timeline of My Healing Journey: A Body Reclaimed from Rash to Resilience

At one point, I didn't even know what "feeling good" meant anymore. I just knew I didn't want to live like I had been living. And now?

“I wake up clear, light, strong, and proud of what my body can do.” – Jackie

The following snapshots aren’t about before-and-after bodies. They’re about before-and-after beliefs.

Every photo tells part of the story, fatigue, resilience, peace, and joy. Each image marks a season of becoming more at home in my own body. “I didn’t just heal my gut. I came back to life.”

Before: Surviving, Not Thriving

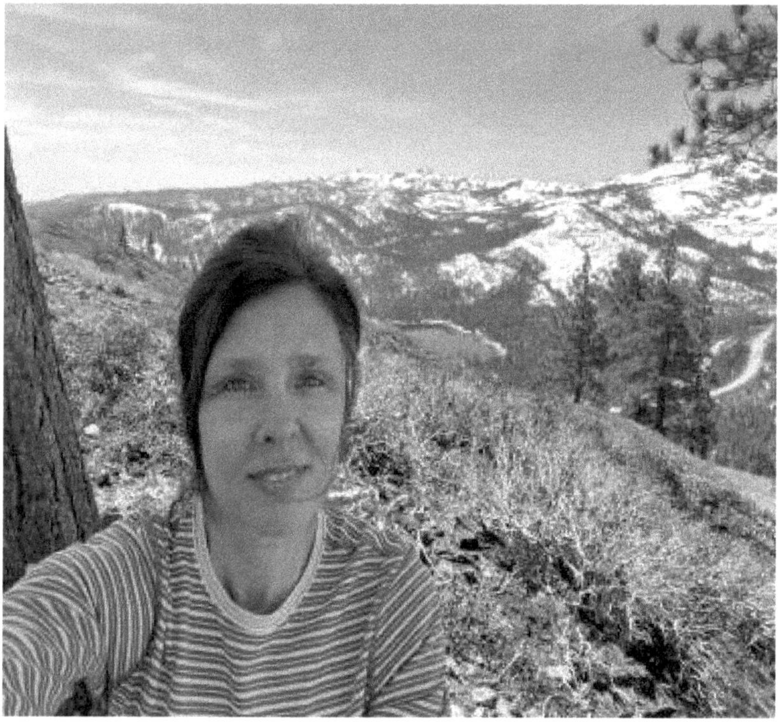

Before I learned about functional medicine, I was living on adrenaline and didn’t know how connected my gut and emotions were. Fatigue, flares, and confusion are all symptoms that are hidden under layers of drive, perfectionism, and survival mode.

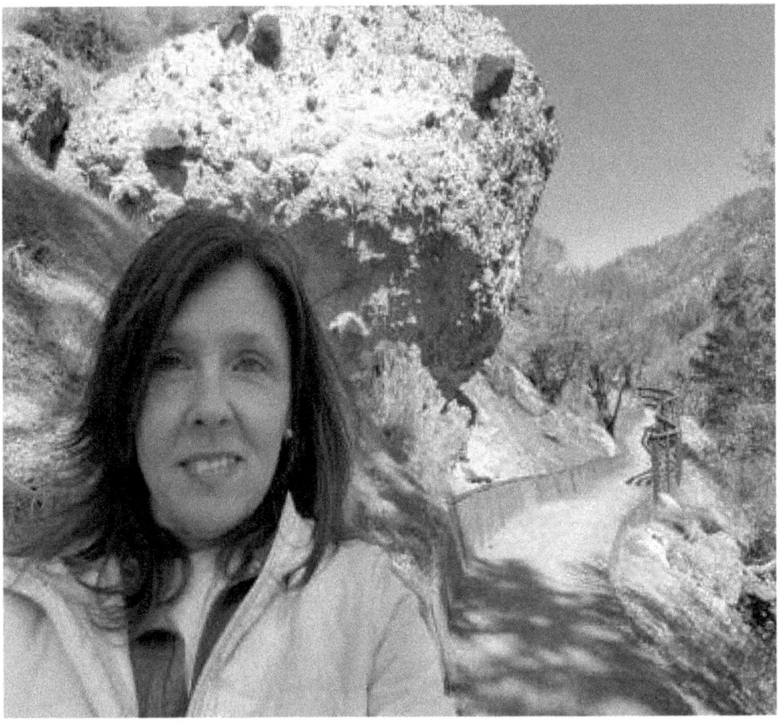

Behind the "smile"? Gut pain, inflammation, and an inner scream for help, silenced by routine and societal norms. Symptoms, fatigue, and emotional overwhelm were constant companions.

During the healing process

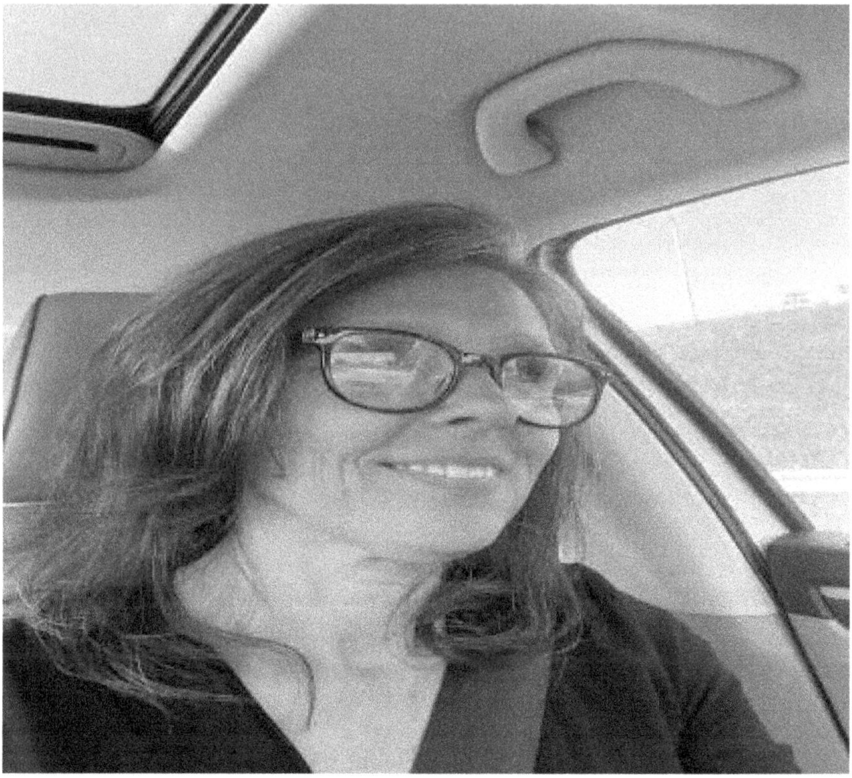

Mid-journey—reconnecting with breathwork, travel, and gentle movement. Active but inflamed, struggling with food, skin, and bloating, knowing there had to be another way.

After: My Gut-Brain Reset

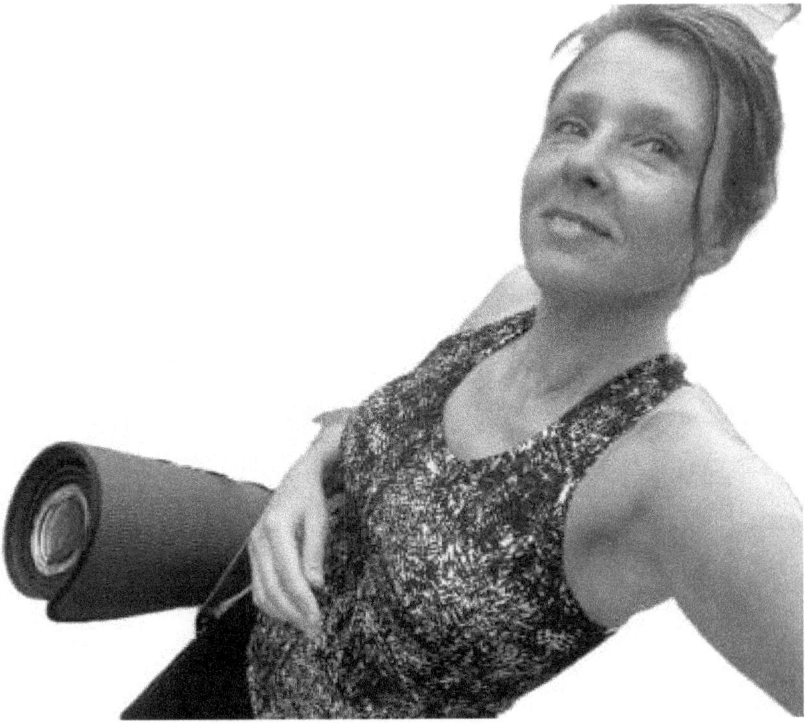

Radiant, resilient, rested. No more "just surviving"—I live each day with energy and intention. Calm. Clear. Confident. No more guessing games. I know how my body works. I trust its wisdom. I've reclaimed my strength. Yoga mat in hand, I walk proud, not because I'm perfect, but because I chose to heal.

These photos are proof that your body can heal when given the right support, space, and belief.

Five Key Strategies for Maintaining the Gut-Brain Loop

Your gut and brain are in constant conversation. So how do you keep peace between them?

1. Use symptoms as signals, not shame.

- Your body is a biofeedback machine. A flare-up isn't failure, it's communication.
- Ask: What changed this week? Sleep? Stress? Food?
- Let your body speak. Don't silence it—tune in.

2. Balance your nervous system first. You can't out-supplement a life of chronic stress.

- Keep up your yin yoga, meditation, or breathwork.
- Walk in nature (daily if possible).
- Protect your evening—it's sacred time for healing.

"The parasympathetic nervous system is the master key for digestion, detox, and repair." – Functional Medicine Principle

3. Honor your gut's daily rhythm.

- Space meals 3–4 hours apart to allow the migrating motor complex to function.
- Stick to three real meals, no grazing.
- Prioritize protein + fiber + fat for satiation, stability, and smooth motility.
- Stay hydrated (clean water like AquaTru is gold).

4. Check in monthly: The "Vital Five".

Each month, do a quick personal audit:

- Bowel Movements—Daily, smooth, easy?
- Skin—Clear, rash free, hydrated?

- Mood—Less reactive, more grounded?
- Energy—Steady across the day?
- Sleep—Falling and staying asleep?

If one is off, that's your clue. Revisit protocol tools or make small adjustments.

Prevention is the sweet spot where traditional medicine and functional medicine work together. Your doctor helps ensure you are safe and supported, while your lifestyle practices help keep you vibrant, stable, and resilient between visits.

5. Live in alignment, not perfection.

You'll travel. Eat cake. Stay up late. That's life. What matters is your baseline—your default state. Let your default be:

Trust over fear
Rituals over routines
Food as fuel, not control
Nature as your gym
Joy as your medicine

Some Thoughts on "Falling Off"

You're going to have setbacks. You're human. Just remember: you've built a toolkit (and you know how to use it!). You are never "starting over."

"I don't reset because I failed. I reset because I respect my body enough to listen."

Gut Maintenance Toolkit (Post-Healing Phase)

- Probiotic (Seed)
  - Why it matters: Supports microbial resilience
  - Frequency: Daily

- Magnesium Glycinate

- Why it matters: Promotes sleep, calm, and healthy digestion/motility
  - Frequency: PM

- Digestive Bitters
  - Why it matters: Aids stomach acid production, readies your digestive system for a meal
  - Frequency: Before meals

- Omega-3 / Collagen
  - Why it matters: Reduces inflammation and aids tissue repair
  - Frequency: Daily

- Food Journal (short term)
  - Why it matters: Tracks possible food triggers and flare patterns in your body
  - Frequency: As needed

- Movement & Breath
  - Why it matters: Regulates the nervous system and supports detox pathways (like your lymphatic system)
  - Frequency: 5× per week

- Vitamin D + K2
  - Why it matters: Strengthens immunity, bones, and gut integrity
  - Frequency: Daily

Retesting and Recalibrating

If you're feeling off after 6–12 months, consider (on your own or with your health practitioner):

- Retesting for food sensitivities
- Revisiting stool or micronutrient testing

- Checking hormones or stress markers (DHEA, cortisol)
- A seasonal reset (see next chapter)

Coming Up Next

In the next chapter, you'll learn about the impact of having mold in your environment and what you can—and must—do about it.

Reminder: *You are not broken. You are brilliant. And the gut you healed isn't just a health achievement—it's your home.*

Chapter 14: The Mold & Toxin Trap

When Hidden Exposure Keeps You Sick

Before I understood mold, I thought a little dust and a leaky basement were harmless. That was until I stayed in that charming cottage in Maine that I mentioned in chapter 9. Within 24 hours, I felt off:

- Brain fog
- Headache
- Sore throat
- Deep fatigue

At first, I chalked it up to travel, but by day two, I saw it, black mold lining the corners of the bathroom ceiling. Ugh! The symptoms weren't in my head—they were in my cells.

When I returned home, I couldn't shake it. I felt off, my sinuses were inflamed, and my nervous system felt like it was buzzing. The team at the UltraWellness Center ordered a urine mycotoxin test, and it all clicked.

Mold: The Fungus That Fights Back

Mold is more than an ugly nuisance; it's an invisible enemy. When spores settle in damp environments like basements, bathrooms, or behind walls, they can make you sick—really sick.

Some common symptoms of mold exposure are:

- Persistent fatigue
- Brain fog or memory loss
- Anxiety and mood swings
- Sinus congestion or nosebleeds
- Rashes or skin itching
- Heightened food sensitivities

- Hormonal imbalances
- Unexpected allergic reactions

Mold and *Candida*: Toxic Twin Flames

Most doctors treat *Candida* and mold separately, but the truth is, they're toxic teammates. Mold makes the immune system weaker, and *Candida* flares up. Detox can't keep up with *Candida*, and mold gets stronger. Together, they exhaust your nervous system and gut repair systems.

This is why you need antifungal nutrition, mold detox, and support for your nervous system all at once.

My doctors were there to help and got the answers we needed for the healing to begin.

Is Your Environment Keeping You Sick?

You can eat perfectly and still feel sick if your environment is inflamed. Here's how I knew something bigger was going on:

- I'd flare up in certain buildings.
- My symptoms worsened after traveling.
- A musty smell in my home triggered headaches.

Eventually, I realized I wasn't just reacting to food. I was reacting to the air.

Common Signs You May Be Living with Mold

- Musty smells that never fully go away
- Window condensation or water damage
- Air vents with visible dust or streaks
- Symptoms that improve when you leave the house
- Chronic sinus infections or wheezing

The Emotional Impact of Mold

Mold messes with more than your sinuses. It steals your clarity and confidence. You start questioning your own body, doubting your intuition, and wondering why no one believes you. Here's the truth:

You're not crazy, you're inflamed.

You're not too sensitive, you're attuned.

Mold can trigger grief, depression, fear, and even PTSD-like symptoms. Dealing with mold is not just a detox; it's an emotional rebuild.

Real Gut-Healing Story: Sarah – "The Classroom That Made Me Sick"

Sarah, 42, loved her job as a teacher. But every year, when spring came, so did the sinus infections, migraines, and body aches. Her doctor said it was allergies. She wasn't so sure.

The moldy ceiling tiles in her classroom were eventually replaced, but her symptoms lingered. That's when she stumbled across mold toxicity and mycotoxin testing.

Her urine test showed elevated ochratoxin A and trichothecenes—two potent mold toxins.

After remediation at home, switching schools, and adding binders plus glutathione to her routine, Sarah felt clearer. Her joint pain faded, her mood lifted, and she finally felt like herself again.

"I was gas lighting myself for years. Now I listen to what my body is trying to say."

Testing for Mold Exposure

Here a few tests you can use to find out if you have mold in your environment.

- Urine Mycotoxin Test
  - Labs: Great Plains, Vibrant Wellness
  - Looks for: ochratoxin A, aflatoxins, trichothecenes
- ERMI or HERTSMI Home Tests
  - Dust collection to identify mold species and levels
- VCS (Visual Contrast Sensitivity) Test
  - Quick online tool to check for mold-related neurotoxicity

If you find mold:

- Hire certified mold inspectors (IICRC or ACAC certified).
- Use independent labs (not just what remediation companies suggest).
- Address the source first—leaks, dampness, ventilation.

Mold remediation is *not* a DIY project. Hire professionals, protect yourself during removal, and follow up with air-quality testing.

Detox Support after Mold Exposure

Here's what helped me safely move toxins out, without crashing:

Foundational Supports:

- Binders: activated charcoal, GI Detox, bentonite clay
- Glutathione
- Infrared sauna: two to three times per week

- Nasal rinses: Xlear or CitriDrops for mold biofilms
- Liver support: castor oil packs, dandelion tea, dry brushing

My Top Tools:

- HEPA air filter (AirDoctor, IQAir)
- Safe skincare, home, and cleaning products
- Daily grounding, hydration, and rebounding (mini-trampoline)

A Final Reminder

If you've hit a plateau, consider your environment. Mold is stealthy and can wreak havoc on your health. You don't need to panic, but you do need to pay attention. You can't out-supplement your surroundings.

Coming Up Next

In chapter 15, I'll give you a powerful, actionable roadmap to help you maintain your results and keep evolving.

Chapter 15: Your 30-Day Gut-Mind Reset Plan

Real Healing. Real Results. One Day at a Time.

Healing is not an event. It's a process—and often a nonlinear one. But when you give your body the right conditions, it knows how to come back into balance. This 30-day plan is the beginning. It's about building momentum. This is the part of the book—where I was not that long ago—where you move from learning to living.

What Makes This Different

This isn't a cookie-cutter cleanse. It's a foundational, functional-medicine–informed protocol built from real results and real life. Some things may be part of your healing and others not as much.

You'll be using principles from:

- Anti-*Candida* + gut repair nutrition
- Nervous system regulation
- Breathwork, movement, and detoxification
- My exact supplement strategies
- Food sensitivity awareness (game changer)
- A daily rhythm that restores the body's natural intelligence
- Mitochondrial and detoxification support

The Reset Promise

By the end of this 30-day plan, your gut will be more balanced, your energy more stable, your mind clearer—and your relationship with your body more whole.

Whether you've been struggling for years or are just starting your journey, this is a blueprint that meets you where you are and moves you forward.

This is not the end. This is your new beginning.

Healing Focus by Week

Each week of healing has a specific focus for restoring your body:

Week 1: Gut reboot: inflammation reduction + elimination of triggers

Week 2: Stabilizing blood sugar and rebalancing the microbiome

Week 3: Supporting detox pathways and restoring the nervous system

Week 4: Integration improving sleep, balancing hormone rhythms, and sustaining long-term support

Daily Healing Rhythm

This daily rhythm mirrors and supports your body's natural cycles of energy, digestion, cleansing, and emotional healing.

Morning

- Wake slowly (no phone first 20 minutes)
- 8 oz warm lemon water (with pinch of sea salt)
- Deep breathing or gratitude journaling (5 minutes)
- Gut-supportive breakfast
- Supplements: Probiotic, magnesium, motility activator (if advised)

Midday

- Walk or gentle movement before lunch
- Gut-boosting lunch
- Bitters before meal, digestive enzymes if tolerated
- Mid-afternoon pause: 10-minute meditation or rest

Evening

- Warming dinner with grounding foods like roasted root vegetables, baked salmon with lemon, drizzled in ghee butter or olive oil, warm broth-based soups.
- Technology off 1 hour before bed
- Herbal tea + magnesium glycinate
- Reflective journaling or light stretching
- Optional: Epsom salt bath or castor oil pack 1–2x/week

Weekly Meal Strategy

Rotate your proteins, vary your vegetables, and stick to low-sugar, anti-inflammatory foods. Include:

- Cooked cruciferous veggies daily
- 1–2 servings of healthy fat per meal
- Lean protein or plant-based options
- Minimal fruit: green apples, grapefruit, berries
- No gluten, dairy, added sugar, or alcohol

Supplement Snapshot (Modify Based on Guidance)

Following is the strategic supplement routine I used during my healing.

Gut Repair

Supplement: L-Glutamine
Notes: 2–5 g AM/PM

Fungal Balance

Supplement: Caprylic acid or oregano
Notes: 1–2 capsules per day

Enzyme Support

Supplement: Digestive enzymes
Notes: Take with meals

Motility

Supplement: Motility activator
Notes: Nighttime only

Mineral Support

Supplement: Magnesium
Notes: AM/PM

Probiotics

Supplement: Seed
Notes: Daily, away from food

Binder Cycling

Supplement: Activated charcoal or GI Detox
Note: Use 30 days on, 7 days off (hydration + fiber intake)

Note: Always consult with your practitioner before starting new supplements.

Functional Lab Testing for Long-Term Help

You don't have to guess, when you can test. Lab work offers powerful feedback so you can stop wondering and worrying what's happening with your body. When done routinely, it helps you stay ahead of imbalances.

- Every six months (while actively healing)
- Once a year (for maintenance and prevention)

For me, it helps knowing I have a team looking out for my best interests and helping me get to the bottom of what's going on and what might be to come.

Tests to Discuss with Your Practitioner

- GI-MAP or stool analysis (microbiome + inflammation)
- Organic Acids Test (OAT) for detox + mitochondrial markers
- Hormone Panels (e.g., DUTCH)
- Food sensitivity (IgG testing)
- Nutrient panels (B vitamins, magnesium, omega-3s)

Questions to Ask Your Functional Practitioner

- What patterns are showing up—even if the test is "normal"?
- How do my gut and hormone results connect?
- Which markers should we recheck in 3–6 months?
- Which supplements are still necessary, and which can I rotate or pause?

Mindset Tools for the Journey

"The gut heals when the nervous system feels safe."

This plan isn't just about what you eat. It's about how you live. Symptoms aren't setbacks—they're signals. They're how the body asks for attention, not punishment.

Daily reflections to try:

How did I take care of myself today?
What food made me feel the most alive today?
What emotion might my symptoms be signaling to me?
Where can I add rest or nourishment tomorrow?

Check in with yourself often. Getting healthy is a lot of work. Be there for yourself now.

Gut Tools for the Journey

- Gut-Safe Grocery List: free download at www.forwardthinkerwellness.com
- Symptom Tracker: create using template format below
- Meal Templates: in chapter 17
- Supplement Planner: examples in previous chapter (always consult with your primary doctor)
- Healing Mindset Prompts: don't do this alone, consider hiring a wellness coach
- Progress Journal Pages: create your own journal or get the companion guide *From Soil to Soul: Rooted & Renewed™* and monitor your health journey

Gut Reset Progress Tracker

Use this 12-week tracker to observe patterns in your energy, digestion, cravings, and mood. Rate each category weekly using circles (❍) or color codes to indicate low → high improvement.

Watch for these common milestones:

- **Weeks 1–2**: Fewer sugar cravings, more awareness of emotional triggers
- **Weeks 3–4**: Improved bowel regularity, better sleep
- **Weeks 5–6**: Increased mental clarity, less histamine reaction
- **Weeks 7–8**: Hormonal regulation, skin clarity, reduced bloating
- **Weeks 9–12**: Emotional breakthroughs, consistent energy, more intuitive eating

Week 1

Energy: ❍❍❍❍

Digestion: ❍❍❍❍

Cravings: ❍❍❍❍

Mood: ❍❍❍❍

Notes: Example – Added lemon water AM.

Week 2

Energy: ❍❍❍❍

Digestion: ❍❍❍❍

Cravings: ❍❍❍❍

Mood: ❍❍❍❍

Notes:

Week 3

Energy: ❍❍❍❍

Digestion: ❍❍❍❍

Cravings: ❍❍❍❍

Mood: ❍❍❍❍

Notes:

Week 4

Energy: ❍❍❍❍

Digestion: ❍❍❍❍

Cravings: ❍❍❍❍

Mood: ❍❍❍❍

Notes:

30-Day Reflection

- What shifted (energy, mood, skin, digestion)?
- What will you keep doing?
- What surprised you?
- What are you ready to reintroduce, if anything?

Week 5–6

Energy: ❍❍❍❍

Digestion: ❍❍❍❍

Cravings: ❍❍❍❍

Mood: ❍❍❍❍

Notes:

Week 7–8

Energy: ❍❍❍❍

Digestion: ❍❍❍❍

Cravings: ❍❍❍❍

Mood: ❍❍❍❍

Notes:

Week 9–10

Energy: ❍❍❍❍

Digestion: ❍❍❍❍

Cravings: ❍❍❍❍

Mood: ❍❍❍❍

Notes:

Week 11–12

Energy: ❍❍❍❍

Digestion: ❍❍❍❍

Cravings: ❍❍❍❍

Mood: ❍❍❍❍

Notes:

Tip: Healing isn't just about getting rid of symptoms; it's also about how you deal with them when they do show up. Be kind to yourself—that's half the battle.

Final Word for This Chapter

You're not just following a plan. You're building a life. One that will hold more quality and will serve you well in the long run.

Coming Up Next

In the next chapter, we'll talk food—what to buy and how to prep it so you can make your healing lifestyle sustainable.

Chapter 16: Gut-Staples for Real Life

Real Food: Your First and Forever Medicine

During my healing journey, food wasn't just fuel, it was medicine (still is). But more than that, it was a mindset. Healing meant creating a space where nourishment felt simple, peaceful, and doable on even the busiest days. This chapter is about readiness—how to stock your kitchen, simplify your choices, and stay balanced wherever life takes you.

Kitchen Philosophy

Your kitchen is your first pharmacy. Healing starts with what you bring home from the grocery store, as well as what you choose not to. So choose wisely.

Here's what I live by:

- Keep it real. If it comes from the earth, not a factory, you're halfway there.
- Reduce sugar (this is a big one). Choose food that stabilizes, not spikes.
- Cook a few basics each week, in batches if you can, so you can rest instead of scramble.
- Clean space = calm body. Clutter in the kitchen often mirrors stress in the gut.
- Choose progress over perfection.

Pantry + Refrigerator Staples

You want to be able to open your pantry or your fridge and feel calm, not confused. Here are the quiet, real food heroes that keep a healing lifestyle doable:

Healthy fats: coconut oil, olive oil, avocado oil

Proteins: wild salmon, sardines, organic eggs, grass-fed meats

Plant fiber: broccoli, cauliflower, kale, Brussels sprouts

Flavor + function: garlic, ginger, turmeric, lemon, apple cider vinegar

Mineral support: sea salt, herbs, dark leafy greens

Snacks that travel: nuts, seeds, coconut flakes, chia, flax, hemp

Hydration helpers: herbal teas (dandelion, peppermint, nettle), electrolyte mixes

Comfort bases: bone or veggie broth, canned lentils, frozen veggies

Real-World Kitchen Habits

- **Prep once, eat easy.** Wash produce, cook proteins, and make a few sauces or dressings each week.
- **Love the labels.** Write the date and a note like "Tuesday soup." It helps future-you stay organized.
- **Five-minute reset.** At night, wipe counters, refill your water filter, set out lemon and sea salt for morning. Basically, set yourself up for success.
- **Simplify cookware.** It's nice to have a chef's kitchen, or, if you're like me, you can get by with just a blender, a cast-iron pan, mason jars, and a good knife.
- **Soothe your senses.** Play music while you cook. Light a candle. Healing food absorbs good energy too.

Behind the Plan

Every kitchen tells a story. Mine began in survival mode, with jars of supplements, half-eaten avocados, and endless stacks of dishes.

Over time, however, it became a sanctuary. The same counter that once held chaos now holds intention: a mug of lemon water, a cutting board, a vase of herbs, a reminder that simplicity heals. And I buy as I go, which helps keep me honest.

Additional Healing Habits

- Keep a "grab-and-go" basket by the door with tea bags, supplements, and protein packs.
- Try freezing lemon slices and bone broth cubes for quick nutrient boosts!
- Put plants in your kitchen. Fresh air is good for digestion too.
- Use glass instead of plastic for food storage.
- Choose filtered water—your gut's best friend.
- Keep a small journal in a drawer for gratitude or meal notes. (I take pictures and have a "food folder" on my desktop.)
- Do light stretches while the water boils or the oven preheats. Movement keeps energy flowing.

Reflection Prompt

How do you make your kitchen look like the life you're creating instead of the one you're leaving behind?

Coming Up Next

If you're wondering what to do with all these ingredients, don't worry—Chapter 17 gives you all-day recipes your body and your tastebuds will love.

Chapter 17: Get the Fungus Outta Here

Healing Recipes from the "Gut Kitchen"

Real food. Real healing. Recipes to help me reclaim my health—one bite at a time.

These recipes aren't "perfect"—but they're real, and they came from real places:

- A trip to Paris, steaming broccoli with the hotel room's coffee maker
- A New York City train ride with homemade snacks
- A beach in Saint Martin, sipping lemon water and journaling
- A retreat in Mexico—meditation and peace at last

They came from late-night cravings, early-morning resets, and long train trips across the country with a lemon in one hand and protein balls in the other! They were born in moments of fatigue, creativity, and fierce determination. Most of all, they were built for real life—food that supports your gut, soothes your mind, and makes healing feel like nourishment, not punishment.

These recipes are just a "taste" of what's to come. Stay tuned for *The Internal Fungus Among Us Kitchen: 30 Days of Gut-friendly Meals!*

Anti-Fungal Power Bowl

Base:

- Steamed cauliflower rice or roasted spaghetti squash

Toppings:

- Wild salmon or tempeh
- Kale wilted in coconut oil

- Avocado slices
- Sauerkraut (if tolerated)
- Pumpkin seeds + lemon juice

Tip: Blend seeds in a coffee grinder to help with absorption.

Immunity Bone Broth

Ingredients:

- 1 organic chicken carcass, beef bone, or veggie scraps (save scraps in the freezer)
- 2 tbsp apple cider vinegar
- Chopped onion, garlic, carrot, celery
- Seaweed, ginger, herbs

Directions: Simmer 12–24 hours. Strain. Sip warm.

Lemon-Garlic Detox Soup

Why It Heals: Garlic is a natural antibiotic, while lemon helps the liver get rid of toxins.

Ingredients:

- 1 tbsp coconut oil
- 2 cloves garlic, minced
- ½ onion, chopped
- 1 zucchini and 1 cup cauliflower florets
- 3 cups bone or veggie broth
- Juice of ½ lemon
- Pinch of turmeric and sea salt

Directions: Sauté garlic and onion in coconut oil until fragrant. Add vegetables and broth, simmer 15 minutes. Blend until smooth, then add lemon juice.

Cauliflower Mash with Thyme and Olive Oil

Why It Heals: A clean, low-carb comfort food that won't feed yeast.

Ingredients:

- 2 cups cauliflower florets
- 1 tbsp olive oil
- Pinch of sea salt
- Fresh thyme to taste (grow your thyme at home—fun and easy!)

Directions: Steam cauliflower until tender. Blend or mash with olive oil, salt, and thyme.

Coconut Curry Veggie Bowl

Why It Heals: Coconut and curry both contain antifungal properties.

Ingredients:

- 1 tbsp coconut oil
- ½ can coconut milk
- 1 cup chopped veggies (broccoli, zucchini, kale)
- 1 tsp curry powder + fresh ginger
- a pinch of black pepper (measure with your heart—this is your health journey)

Directions: Sauté veggies in coconut oil with ginger. Add coconut milk and curry powder, then let it simmer 10 minutes. Serve over cauliflower rice.

Apple Cider Vinegar Morning Drink

Why It Heals: Balances pH, improves digestion, and helps break down yeast biofilm.

Ingredients:

- 1 tbsp apple cider vinegar
- 1 cup warm water
- Dash of cinnamon or cinnamon stick

Directions: Stir all ingredients together and drink slowly before breakfast.

Zucchini Noodles with Lemon-Basil Pesto

Why It Heals: No grains, no sugar—just fresh herbs and fats that fight inflammation.

Ingredients:

- 2 zucchini, spiraled
- 1 cup basil leaves
- 1 clove garlic
- ¼ cup olive oil
- Juice of half a lemon
- Sea salt to taste

Directions: Blend basil, garlic, olive oil, and lemon into pesto. Toss with zucchini noodles and top with sea salt.

Garlic-Rosemary Roasted Chicken

Why It Heals: Protein keeps blood sugar steady, while herbs offer antifungal protection.

Ingredients:

- 4 chicken thighs
- 1 tbsp coconut oil
- 2 cloves garlic, minced
- 1 tbsp fresh rosemary
- Juice of half a lemon

Directions: Preheat oven to 375°F. Rub chicken with oil, garlic, rosemary, and lemon juice. Bake 30–35 minutes until golden brown and cooked through.

Peruvian Chicken (homestyle/family recipe varies)

Why It Heals: one of my unexpected comfort foods during my healing journey. It was simple, flavorful, and naturally aligned with functional medicine principles, offering high-quality protein, bright herbs, and ingredients that supported my gut rather than inflaming it.

Ingredients:

- 1 lb chicken thighs (inexpensive and savory!)
- 1 tsp smoked paprika
- 2 cloves chopped garlic
- 1 tbsp soy sauce (or gluten-free aminos)
- Juice of one lime
- 1 tsp mustard
- 1 tsp honey (omit during a flare-up)
- 1/2 tsp cumin
- 1 tsp oregano (I use fresh and more!)
- 1/2 tsp black pepper
- 3 pinches of sea salt
- 1 tbsp of avocado oil

Directions: In a bowl, mix all ingredients and marinate the chicken in the fridge for about an hour. Bring frying pan to medium-high temp, then blacken chicken to desired color. Finish cooking in oven at 425°F for about 30 minutes. This freezes well, so make a double batch!

Green Goddess Anti-Fungal Smoothie

Why It Heals: Replaces sugary smoothies with nutrients, greens, and fats that are good for your gut.

Ingredients:

- 1 cup coconut milk
- 1 handful spinach + parsley
- ½ avocado
- 1 tbsp flaxseed + 1 tsp coconut oil
- ½ green apple

Directions: Blend all ingredients until smooth and sip slowly to help digestion.

Ginger-Turmeric Healing Elixir

Why It Heals: Fights inflammation and pathogens while soothing the liver.

Ingredients:

- 1 cup water
- ½ inch fresh ginger, sliced
- ½ tsp turmeric powder
- Pinch of black pepper

Directions: Simmer ingredients in water for 10 minutes. Strain and sip warm.

Cabbage and Carrot Stir-Fry

Why It Heals: Cruciferous veggies detox estrogen and mold byproducts, as well as provide fiber and prebiotics.

Ingredients:

- 1 tbsp coconut oil
- 2 cups shredded cabbage
- 1 cup shredded carrots
- 1 tsp tamari or coconut aminos
- Sesame or flax seeds to sprinkle on top

Directions: Sauté veggies in coconut oil for 5–7 minutes. Add tamari or aminos, stir, and sprinkle with sesame or flax seeds.

I have eaten this for breakfast, there are no rules about not eating lunch for breakfast!

Savory Seed Crackers

Why It Heals: Replaces yeast-feeding bread with fiber-rich, steadying crunch.

Ingredients:

- ¼ cup flax seeds
- ¼ cup chia seeds
- ¼ cup pumpkin seeds
- ½ cup water
- Sea salt and herbs to taste

Directions: Mix seeds and water, let sit 10 minutes. Spread mixture thinly on parchment and bake at 300°F for 30–40 minutes until crisp.

The first time I made these, it was a mess—the crackers were fat and crumbly. I ate them anyway and refined the recipe. If you don't get it right the first time, try again!

Lemon-Ginger Poached Salmon

Why It Heals: Omega-3 fats reduce inflammation and improve gut-lining integrity.

Ingredients:

- 2 salmon fillets (wild caught, local if available)
- 2 cups water or broth
- 3 lemon slices
- 3 ginger slices

- Sea salt to taste

Directions: Simmer salmon with lemon, ginger, and salt for 10–12 minutes or until it flakes.

Coconut-Cinnamon “Sweet Fix” Bites

Why It Heals: Satisfies cravings without feeding yeast.

Ingredients:

- ½ cup coconut flakes
- 2 tbsp coconut oil
- 1 tsp cinnamon
- A few drops stevia or monk fruit if using unsweetened coconut

Directions: Mix ingredients, shape into balls, and chill in fridge until firm.

Once the gut is cleared, it’s time to rebuild. These recipes are designed to restore strength, nourish the microbiome, and bring joy back to the table. They’re anti-inflammatory, nutrient-rich, and deeply comforting—because healing should also taste like home.

Hearty Lentil Veggie Stew

This cozy stew was born on a rainy night when all I wanted was something simple, grounding, and real.

Why It Heals: Lentils are rich in fiber and minerals that help repair the gut lining while supporting steady blood sugar.

Ingredients:

- 1 tbsp olive oil
- 1 small onion, chopped
- 2 carrots, diced

- 1 cup lentils (rinsed), or canned if you're on the go
- 4 cups veggie broth, or bone broth for extra protein
- 1 tsp turmeric
- Sea salt, pepper, and herbs to taste

Directions: Sauté onion and carrots until soft. Add lentils, broth, and spices. Simmer 25–30 minutes until tender. Serve warm and breathe deeply.

Sweet Potato Turmeric Bowl

The colors alone make you feel better—golden, grounding, and alive.

Why It Heals: Sweet potatoes feed beneficial bacteria, and turmeric calms inflammation.

Ingredients:

- 1 sweet potato, cubed and roasted
- 1 cup sauteed spinach or kale
- 1 tbsp tahini or olive oil drizzle
- 1 tsp turmeric + pinch of black pepper

Directions:

Arrange sweet potatoes and greens in a bowl. Sprinkle turmeric and pepper and drizzle with tahini. Enjoy slowly, grounding in each bite.

Wild Salmon with Lemon-Dill Sauce

This recipe reminds me of New England summers—light, simple, and perfectly balanced.

Why It Heals: Rich in omega-3 fatty acids to reduce inflammation and restore gut-brain harmony.

Ingredients:

- 2 wild salmon fillets
- 1 tbsp olive oil
- Juice of ½ lemon
- 1 tbsp fresh dill
- Sea salt and black pepper

Directions: Pan-sear salmon in olive oil until lightly golden. Top with lemon juice and fresh dill. Serve with steamed greens or cauliflower rice.

Carrot-Ginger Soup

A gentle, soothing blend for digestion and emotional calm—like sunshine in a bowl. Great for fall but perfect anytime of the year.

Why It Heals: Ginger and carrots reduce bloating, support bile flow, and restore digestive fire.

Ingredients:

- 1 tbsp coconut oil
- 3 carrots, chopped
- 1 inch fresh ginger, sliced
- 3 cups veggie broth
- Sea salt to taste

Directions: Sauté carrots and ginger in coconut oil. Add broth and simmer until soft. Blend until creamy. Sip warm and let your system rest.

Warm Quinoa Omega Bowl

Perfect for chilly mornings or gentle resets after travel—soft, warm, and nourishing.

Why It Heals: Quinoa provides complete protein and prebiotic fiber to fuel microbiome repair.

Ingredients:

- ½ cup quinoa
- 1 cup coconut or almond milk
- 1 tsp cinnamon
- 1 tsp coconut oil
- Optional: berries or stewed apples

Directions: Simmer quinoa in milk until fluffy. Stir in cinnamon and coconut oil. Top with warm fruit and gratitude.

Gut-Soothing Buddha Bowl

This bowl became my travel go-to—vibrant, easy, and endlessly customizable.

Why It Heals: Combines plant fiber, protein, and healthy fats to stabilize blood sugar and mood, healing from the inside out.

Ingredients:

- Base: cauliflower rice or quinoa
- Protein: wild salmon, tempeh, or eggs (if tolerated)
- Veggies: kale, cucumber, shredded carrots
- Toppings: avocado, seeds, and tahini drizzle

Directions: Assemble all ingredients in a bowl. Top with seeds and tahini drizzle. Pause before eating—notice the colors, feel the gratitude.

Coconut-Lime Chicken

Bright and refreshing, this dish is a post-cleanse favorite—light yet deeply satisfying.

Why It Heals: Coconut fights microbes while lime stimulates digestion and adds a burst of vitamin C.

Ingredients:

- 2 chicken breasts
- ½ cup coconut milk
- Juice of 1 lime
- 1 clove garlic, minced
- Sea salt and cilantro to taste

Directions: Marinate chicken in coconut milk, lime, and garlic for 30 minutes. Grill or pan-sear until cooked through. Top with fresh cilantro and lime zest.

Citrus Glow Dressing

A simple dressing that turns any salad or bowl into a detox boost for your liver.

Why It Heals: Lemon and olive oil support bile flow and detox while brightening flavor naturally.

Ingredients:

- Juice of 1 lemon
- 2 tbsp olive oil
- 1 tsp apple cider vinegar
- Pinch of sea salt and black pepper

Directions: Whisk or shake all ingredients in a jar. Drizzle over roasted veggies or greens.

Reishi-Cacao Evening Latte

A warm hug in a mug—this became my nighttime ritual for unwinding and restoring.

Why It Heals: Reishi mushroom calms the nervous system; cacao soothes mood and cravings.

Ingredients:

- 1 cup almond or coconut milk
- 1 tsp cacao powder
- ½ tsp reishi powder
- Pinch cinnamon and vanilla

Directions: Warm milk, then whisk in powders and spices. Sip slowly and let your system shift toward rest.

Matcha Coconut Energy Bites

For long days or travel, these bites are clean fuel—no crash, just calm energy.

Why It Heals: Matcha provides steady caffeine, while coconut supports metabolism and focus.

Ingredients:

- ½ cup shredded coconut
- 2 tbsp coconut oil
- 1 tsp matcha powder
- 1 tbsp ground flaxseed
- Stevia or monk fruit to taste

Directions: Mix ingredients and roll into small bites. Chill until firm. Take them wherever life leads.

Reflection Prompts

Which foods make you feel clean, serene, and in charge—not restricted, but restored?

Which meals make you feel most at home in your body?

What does nourishment mean to you now?

Chapter 18: Final Words

You Are the Healer You've Been Waiting For

There was a time when I thought I'd never feel whole again. My energy was gone. My gut was inflamed. My emotions were raw. My future felt blurry.

I searched everywhere—for answers, protocols, quick fixes, any fix, and miracle supplements...

What I found was something deeper: Healing was never outside of me. It was always within.

You've just completed a journey through functional healing—body, mind, and soul. You've explored the gut-brain axis, emotional detox, antifungal nutrition, nervous system repair, and spiritual resilience. You are a "rock star." And more than anything, you've learned to trust your body's wisdom. This isn't goodbye. This is the beginning.

You Are Now Your Own Expert

You will still consult practitioners. You may try new protocols or therapies. But now, everything runs through a new filter: your intuition.

You've learned what nourishes you. You've discovered what drains you. You know what your body sounds like—because you've begun to listen. That's everything.

Healing Creates Ripples

You didn't do this just for yourself. Your healing will touch your partner, your family, your community, your children, and even people you'll never meet.

When we show up whole, we give others permission to do the same. So pass it on. Share what worked for you and didn't. Offer grace and a listening ear when someone is still stuck. Be a lighthouse, not a lecture.

A Sacred Thank You

Thank you for walking this path with me. For trusting these words. For showing up—even when it was hard.

I pray you carry forward a deeper belief in your body's design, your nervous system's resilience, and your soul's calling.

Let this be your reminder: "You are not broken. You are becoming."

You've learned the tools. You've done the work.

And now... Go live.

With deep love,

Jackie

Afterword

I wrote most of this book between two sacred spaces. One was a quiet farm on a hill, where wildlife wandered freely and the wide fields asked me to slow down, breathe deeper, and listen inward in a way that felt ancient and necessary. The mornings there were soft, the kind that invite honesty. Healing always felt closer on that land.

The other was a barn by the sea, a beautifully restored space with high wooden beams and a quietness that felt almost holy. Something about being near the water softened my mind. The tide kept its own steady rhythm just beyond the walls, and the ocean air carried a clarity I could feel even from inside. Thoughts loosened, ideas opened, and creativity flowed as if the coastline itself was guiding my hand. It was a place where writing felt effortless, honest, and alive.

These places were my sanctuaries. They steadied me, softened me, and held my becoming. They brought these pages to life.

* * *

Becoming Manifesto

For the woman I am, and the legacy I live

I am no longer living to be chosen

I stand in the center of my own life, not out of reaction, but intention

I do not chase love, validation, or belonging

I cultivate it, I carry it, I anchor it within myself

I have walked through pain and did not stay there

I learned the lesson, integrated the wisdom, and now I lead through how I live

I do not survive, I expand

I do not wait for peace, I build it with every rooted choice I make

I am in transition, not turmoil

I am becoming, and the world is adjusting around me

Even when paths shift or relationships stretch,

I remain connected to who I am, steady in truth, steady in faith, steady in self

I lead with love, grounded in clarity

I am legacy in motion

I am already whole

jMf

7/15/2025

Appendix: Gut-Healing Tools & Resources

A practical toolkit to accompany your healing journey—complete with the functional tests, supplements, spiritual tools, and lifestyle practices mentioned throughout this book. This appendix serves as your go-to healing dashboard: quick-access, printable, and designed to keep your reset simple and sustainable.

For live links, downloads, and updated recommendations, visit
www.forwardthinkerwellness.com.

Daily Gut Reset Checklist

Morning

- 10 minutes of breathwork or quiet reflection
- 16 oz warm lemon water
- Gut-supportive supplements (see protocol)
- Protein-rich breakfast with healthy fats and fiber

Midday

- Anti-inflammatory "build-your-plate"–style lunch
- 10- to 15-minute outdoor walk
- Herbal tea (peppermint, ginger, or fennel)

Evening

- Cooked, grounding dinner
- Magnesium support + Motility Activator (if needed)
- Journaling practice
- Lights dimmed by 9 PM, in bed by 10 PM

Grocery Guide: Gut-Healing Foods to Stock Your Kitchen

- Proteins
  - Organic chicken or turkey
  - Grass-fed beef
  - Wild-caught salmon, cod, sardines
  - Pasture-raised eggs
  - Lentils, chickpeas, black beans (if tolerated)
  - Organic tempeh
  - Clean collagen or bone broth
- Vegetables (choose 8–10 weekly)
  - Zucchini, squash
  - Broccoli, cauliflower, cabbage
  - Spinach, kale, Swiss chard
  - Sweet potatoes, carrots, beets
  - Asparagus, cucumbers, green beans
  - Onions, garlic, leeks (prebiotic powerhouses)
- Fruit (naturally antifungal or low-hypoglycemic)
  - Blueberries
  - Raspberries
  - Green apples
  - Strawberries
  - Lemons, limes
  - Grapefruit (if tolerated)
- Healthy Fats
  - Avocado
  - Extra virgin olive oil
  - Coconut oil
  - Ghee
  - Walnuts
  - Pumpkin seeds

    - Almonds
    - Chia seeds and flax seeds

- Herbs & Spices (anti-inflammatory + gut-healing)
    - Ginger
    - Turmeric
    - Cinnamon
    - Basil, rosemary, thyme
    - Oregano
    - Parsley, cilantro

- Fermented & Functional Foods
    - Sauerkraut
    - Kimchi
    - Coconut yogurt
    - Miso
    - Apple cider vinegar

- Low-Toxin Carbs
    - Quinoa
    - Brown rice
    - Gluten-free oats
    - Cassava tortillas
    - Sweet potatoes

- Gut-Friendly Beverages
    - Herbal teas (ginger, peppermint, chamomile)
    - Green tea
    - Mineral water
    - Electrolytes (clean ingredients only)

- Pantry Essentials
    - Coconut milk
    - Tomato paste, crushed tomatoes
    - Lentils
    - Chickpeas

- Gluten-free pasta
- Clean broth
- Organic spices
- Almond flour

Core Supplement Protocol (Customizable)

Always consult with your healthcare provider before starting supplements.

Morning

- Probiotic (e.g., Seed Daily Synbiotic)
- Magnesium citrate (supports motility)
- Digestive enzymes before meals

Afternoon

- Omega-3 (anti-inflammatory support)
- Curcumin or turmeric (for inflammation)

Evening

- Magnesium glycinate (for sleep and nervous system)
- Motility Activator (if experiencing constipation)
- Adaptogenic support (Ashwagandha or rhodiola)

Functional Labs & Testing

- Wellevate / Fullscript—Access practitioner-recommended tests and protocols at https://fullscript.com
- Mosaic Diagnostics (formerly Great Plains)—Organic acids, mycotoxin, and environmental toxin testing
- Genova Diagnostics—GI Effects stool panel and comprehensive micronutrient test
- Precision Analytical—DUTCH hormone panel

- 3x4 Genetics—Personalized gene-based health insights

All of these specialty labs and functional tests can be accessed through my wellness portal, where I help clients interpret results and create customized next steps.

Suggested Reading + Influences

- *The Ultra Mind Solution*—Mark Hyman, MD
- *The Autoimmune Solution*—Amy Myers, MD
- *The Mind-Gut Connection*—Emeran Mayer, MD
- *Brain Maker*—David Perlmutter, MD
- *The 10-Day Detox Diet*—Mark Hyman, MD

Functional Medicine + Clinical Support

- Hyman, M. (2021). *The Pegan Diet: 21 Practical Principles for Reclaiming Your Health in a Nutritionally Confusing World. Little, Brown Spark.*
- "Institute for Functional Medicine. (n.d.). Root-cause medicine education and practitioner resources." Retrieved November 2025, from https://www.ifm.org
- The UltraWellness Center. (n.d.). Functional medicine practice founded by Dr. Mark Hyman. Retrieved November 2025, from https://www.ultrawellnesscenter.com
- Dr. Mark Hyman, MD's "*10-Day Detox.*" https://drhyman.com/pages/10-day-detox
- Cleveland Clinic Center for Functional Medicine. (n.d.). Integrative care for chronic conditions. Retrieved November 2025, from https://my.clevelandclinic.org/departments/functional-medicine
- National Library of Medicine. (n.d.). National Center for Biotechnology Information (NCBI). Retrieved November 2025, from https://www.ncbi.nlm.nih.gov

- PubMed. (n.d.). Biomedical and life sciences research database. Retrieved November 2025, from https://pubmed.ncbi.nlm.nih.gov

Movement & Embodied Healing Practitioners

- **Jurian Hughes**, Senior Faculty, Kripalu School of Yoga; E-RYT 500, YACEP.
  Website: jurianhughes.com
  YogaDance, movement, ritual, voice, online classes, and retreats
- **Jess Frey**, Lead Faculty, Kripalu; E-RYT 1000.
  Website: kripalu.org/people/jess-frey
  Somatic journaling, yoga, mindful movement, online programs

Resources for Gut-healing Food and Supplements

Seed Health. (n.d.). Seed Probiotic is a clinically proven Synbiotic that helps the gut microbiome. Taken from https://www.seed.com on November 2025.

- AquaTru. (n.d.). Reverse-osmosis water purification systems for home and travel. Retrieved November 2025, from https://www.aquatruwater.com
- Gaia Herbs. (n.d.). Digestive bitters and herbal wellness formulas. Retrieved November 2025, from https://www.gaiaherbs.com
- Pure Encapsulations. (n.d.). Professional-grade nutritional supplements. Retrieved November 2025, from https://www.pureencapsulations.com
- Fullscript. (n.d.). Cortisol Manager – Integrative Therapeutics stress and sleep support (formula available via practitioner portal). Retrieved November 2025, from https://www.fullscript.com
- Hari-Om School of Yoga and Ayurveda. (n.d.). Kitchari Cleanse – Ayurvedic reset for digestive balance.

Retrieved November 2025, from https://www.hari-om.it

- Vital Proteins. (n.d.). Collagen peptides help the joints and gut. From https://www.vitalproteins.com retrieved in November 2025.

Dispensary my Recommended Product Dispensary

Visit my Fullscript Dispensary at www.forwardthinkerwellness.com for professional-grade supplements and my personal wellness faves. (These are compilations of digestive, immunological, and hormone support items that I have put together from my own healing path.)

Filtering Water—I suggest AquaTru Water Systems for clean, toxin-free water. You can order this on my list of suggested products at www.forwardthinkerwellness.com.

Probiotics—I recommend Seed Synbiotic, which is on my list of recommended products at www.forwardthinkerwellness.com, for daily gut support and a balanced microbiome.

Stress, Energy, and Emotional Healing

- Deepak Chopra *21-Day Meditation Series* – www.chopra.com
- Reiki + Yin Yoga – Trained and certified in the Usui lineage and Yin Yoga programs
- Ayurveda Health Certification – Trained and certified with Pragya Gupta, MD

Labs and Specialty Testing

- Genova Diagnostics (GI Effects, NutrEval)

- Wellevate Food Sensitivity Testing – www.wellevate.me
- Great Plains Laboratory (MycoTox)
- Precision Analytical (DUTCH Test)
- 3x4 Genetics – www.3x4genetics.com

All of these specialty labs and functional tests can be accessed through my wellness coaching portal, where I help clients interpret results and design personalized next steps for healing.

To explore personalized testing, supplement support, or gut-healing guidance, visit my wellness portal at www.forwardthinkerwellness.com.

To Continue Your Healing

Visit forwardthinkerwellness.com for new tools, updated protocols, and companion downloads. This appendix is your ongoing invitation to stay connected—body, mind, and spirit.

About the Author

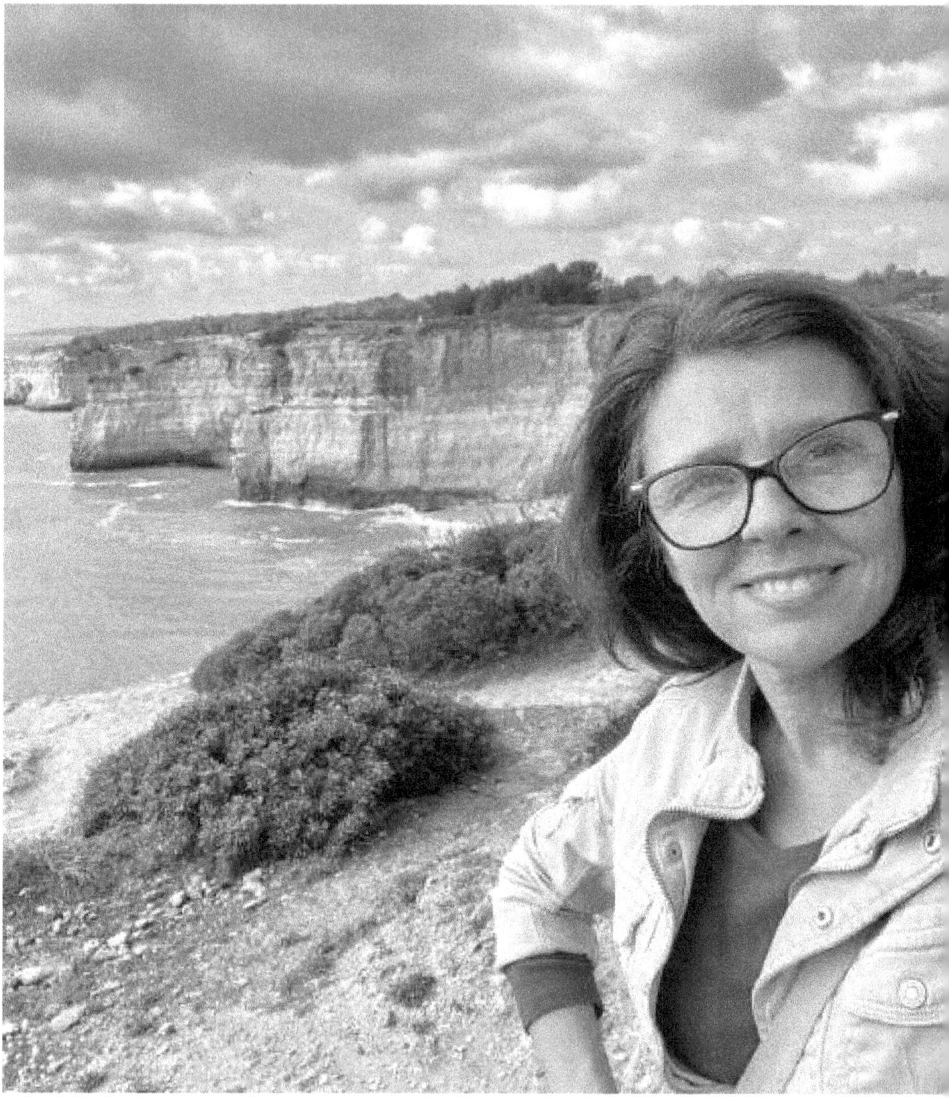

Jackie Frary is a wellness advocate, gut-healing guide, and the heart behind *The Internal Fungus Among Us.* With decades of lived experience navigating candidiasis, IBS, SIBO, food sensitivities, inflammation, and burnout, Jackie transformed her own health through functional medicine, spiritual practice, and a fierce commitment to self-awareness.

After years of "doing everything right" and still feeling wrong, Jackie became her own best advocate. She partnered with practitioners at Mark Hyman MD, UltraWellness Center, completed functional and food sensitivity testing, and designed a personal protocol that reversed symptoms, restored clarity, and reignited joy.

During one of the most emotionally vulnerable phases of her life, Jackie experienced profound grief—losing both her mother and a beloved colleague and friend at the same time, while navigating major life transitions that deepened her healing journey. That chapter of deep loss became a powerful catalyst for healing on an entirely different level.

Jackie holds certifications in Health, Nutrition, and Life Coaching, as well as training in Massage Therapy and Yin Yoga. A Reiki Master and Ayurveda Health Practitioner, she blends functional medicine principles with intuitive, whole-person healing—not to teach perfection, but to help others trust their body's brilliance.

Her approach combines research-backed insight with practical compassion, intuitive healing, and a down-to-earth sense of humor. Jackie has coached others through gut repair, nervous system regulation, and sustainable lifestyle transformation—all from a place of "I've been there."

She lives in New England, loves clean water, mushroom coffee, yoga by the fireplace, and strength training that makes her feel alive. When she's not coaching, writing, or hunting down the cleanest gluten-free granola on Earth, she's helping others come home to themselves.

"Healing is possible. I'm living proof." – Jackie

https://www.forwardthinkerwellness.com

https://www.linkedin.com/in/jackiefrary

https://www.facebook.com/ForwardThinKerWellness

https://www.instagram.com/jfrary00

https://www.forwardthinkerwellness.com

Also by Jackie Frary

After years of unexplained symptoms, tiredness, and anger over "quick fixes," I found out that real healing starts from the inside out—not just in the gut but also in the heart and mind. *The Internal Fungus Among Us* was born from that journey: my search for answers, my partnership with functional medicine, and my faith that the body is designed to heal when given the right environment.

Now, with *From Soil to Soul: Rooted & Renewed*™, a 90-day daily devotional, healing journal, and reflections for whole-body renewal, I help others do the same—one mindful, faith-filled day at a time. My writing combines research and spirituality to help people find balance, strength, and a greater connection to the wisdom of their own bodies.

FROM SOIL
to
SOUL™

Rooted & Renewed

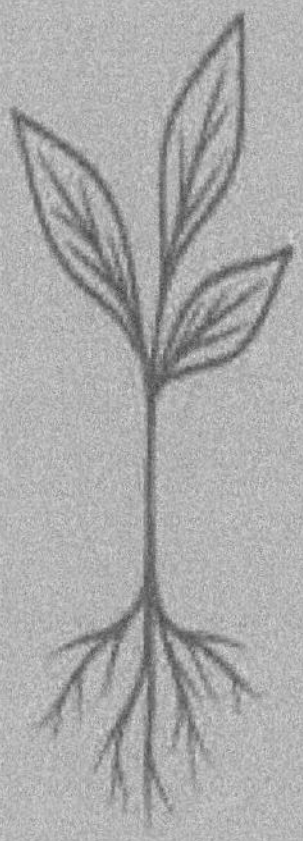

A 90-Day Journal of Healing Devotionals, Reflections & Whole-Body Renewal

Jackie Frary

A daily devotional companion to *The Internal Fungus Among Us*, nurturing spiritual growth, renewal, and mindfulness—for those learning to breathe again, trust the process, and believe that new life can grow from anywhere.

www.ingramcontent.com/pod-product-compliance
Lightning Source LLC
LaVergne TN
LVHW051922051126
851857LV00021B/2105
9798994722329